# WILD MEDICINE
## Autumn and Winter

T0154537

Other books in the series

*Wild Medicine: Spring*
*Wild Medicine: Summer*

# WILD MEDICINE
## Autumn and Winter

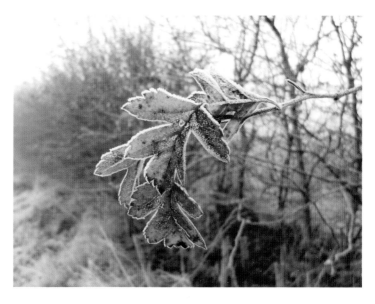

*Ali English*

*Aeon Books*

**Disclaimer**

The intent of this book is solely informational and educational. The information and suggestions in this book are not intended to replace the advice or treatments given by health professionals. The author and publisher have made every effort to present accurate information. However, they shall be neither responsible nor liable for any problem that may arise from information in this book.

First published in 2019 by
Aeon Books Ltd
12 New College Parade
Finchley Road
London NW3 5EP

**British Library Cataloguing in Publication Data**

A C.I.P. for this book is available from the British Library

ISBN:   978–1–91159–768–1

Printed in Great Britain

www.aeonbooks.co.uk

# Contents

# About the Author

Herbalist Ali English has been passionate about herbs from a young age and went on to study herbal medicine at Lincoln University, graduating in 2010 with a BSc (Hons). Since then, she has set up a practice in Lincolnshire that focuses on offering herb walks, workshops and a variety of related services, in which she tries to convey her love of our native herbs and wildflowers to anyone who will listen. *Wild Medicine: Autumn and Winter* is her second book, with many more to follow.

# Acknowledgements

As always, for Matt, for his constant, unstinting support and love; and for my family, as always.

Also for the lovely team at Stella Arden and Associates in Louth & Woodhall Spa, for being excellent cheerleaders!

Many thanks to you all.

# Preface

Welcome to *Wild Medicine: Autumn and Winter*. It is my hope that this series of seasonal books will provide a source of information and kindle a keen delight in the glories of our native plants, both those growing in the hedgerows and those weedy adventurers tucked into nooks and crannies in our own gardens.

At the time of writing this brief introduction, harvest is well underway and the garden is ripening up with all sorts of delicious fruits, nuts and seeds. In the hedgerows, a slow tide of crimson is gradually making its way up the country as the hawthorn berries begin to take on red hues, and later on there will be rosehips garlanding the bushes, ripening slowly until the first frost nips them and renders them perfect for gathering. The first hop strobiles have appeared and will be ready for bringing in sometime in late September, in all their fragrant, resinous glory. I've always spent many happy hours in the autumn gathering in medicines and preparing syrups and tinctures, elixirs and teas, and the scent of rosehip syrup cooking on the hob is synonymous with autumn for me. I added root gathering somewhat later on, about halfway through my formal training as a herbalist, and it is now a cherished part of the yearly routine of gathering and medicine making – and a delightfully messy enterprise that really reintroduces me to the soil every year.

Hopefully this book, which rather arbitrarily divides out a selection of herbs and designates them as autumn and winter herbs, will give you a rough idea of what delights can be gathered and made in the autumn and winter, using herbs, fruits and roots that are available from September through to February. It is by necessity a fairly brief introduction to the subject, but, herbalism being such a vast topic to cover, it may give you a thread to begin following as you commence or continue on your own journey into plant healing. By necessity there will be some plants not covered in this book that can be found in the other two volumes, though I have tried to include some recipes for autumn linked to, for example, the elder tree.

It is my aim that these books will provide hedgerow travel books to tuck into a pocket and take along with you in the warmer seasons and perhaps to inspire and console you through the winter. May they give you many years of enjoyment and help you towards your own deepening friendship with the plants that surround us and give us so much.

Green Blessings!

*North Lincolnshire, 2019*

# Autumn and Winter

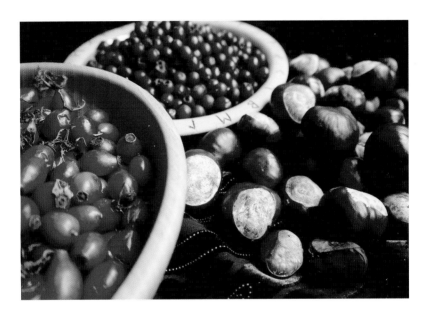

# Introduction:
# gathering and preparing roots, seeds, barks and fruit

Many of the basic skills needed for medicine-making are covered briefly in *Wild Medicine: Summer*, but roots, seeds, barks and fruit require somewhat different preparation and gathering skills. Here is a brief outline of some of the things to remember while gathering and preparing medicines with the ingredients available in autumn and winter.

## Roots

Roots are almost always dug in the autumn and winter, and occasionally (in the case of wood avens, *Geum urbanum*) in early spring before the plant really gets going with the new growth of the year. I tend to recommend that roots are dug in the afternoon and evening, or even at night, when the energy of the plant will be most thoroughly anchored in its roots, a principle that is part of moon gardening and biodynamics. You can even check the planetary ruler of each plant and try to gather on the appropriate days if you want to. I suggest using a garden fork to loosen the soil around the roots thoroughly before you try to unearth the plant itself – remember that some roots, such as burdock, go down an astonishingly long way, so you will need to dig a much deeper hole than you expect to unearth a decent amount of it. In many cases, you can take the side roots of the plants and leave the central rhizome intact. Many plants will happily regrow from a tiny bit of root left in the ground, but do be aware that for most plants the roots are their life force, so show appreciation and respect – and, if you can, sow a few seeds from the plant in its place. Roots of biennial plants, such as burdock and angelica, need to be gathered in the first year, when the plant is in its basal rosette stage before it has flowered, as by the second year any nutrients stored in the roots will have been used to produce the first year's flowers and seeds.

Use a nail brush or an old toothbrush to scrub the surface of any gathered roots thoroughly – this is best done outside, using an outdoor tap if possible, as herb roots can harbour surprising amounts of soil and small passengers, not to mention tiny secondary roots, which will often need to be stripped off and disposed of before preparing the main collection of roots. These threadlike roots have the tendency to block kitchen sinks if prepared indoors. Once the roots are completely clean, chop them into smaller pieces, around 4 mm square, or into thin discs up to 2 mm thick, and use either a dehydrator or an oven on the lowest setting to slowly dry them down for storage. Roots toughen as they dry – if, for example, you dry dandelion roots whole, you will often find them almost impossible to break up again afterwards, as I learned the hard way on one of my first root-gathering expeditions. Once the prepared roots have dried thoroughly and shrunk a bit, they should be ready to store in jars. Remember to label them carefully, with the English and Latin names and the date stored. Roots will usually last quite a bit longer than dried herbs will – up to three years or more, depending on the kind of root. Good-quality dried roots should pack a decent punch of flavour and still have a good colour to them. Angelica and elecampane roots, for example, should still be pungent and punchy; if, though, they have become wishy-washy and bland, it is time to compost them and gather fresh roots.

Roots can also be tinctured fresh, using the strongest alcohol you can obtain (a minimum of 40% proof is ideal, stronger is even better). Simply repeat the first steps of cleaning and finely chopping the roots, leave the surface to dry overnight if you have slightly weaker alcohol, then pack the chopped roots into a Kilner jar, and cover with alcohol, allowing an extra couple of centimetres on top of the herbs, then put the lid on. Leave the whole lot to infuse for at least two weeks – four is often better, as roots will take longer to infuse than leaves do. Remember that the smaller you get the root pieces, the better they will infuse into the alcohol to make a tincture.

# Seeds

Seeds often need to be gathered before they are fully ripe. Gather the top 25 cm (10 in.) of the plant and suspend this upside down in a bundle, with the tops covered by a paper bag or a close-weave cloth bag, fastened in place with an elastic band. As the seeds ripen, they will fall off the plant and land in the bag, after which they can be stored and used as needed. Nettles can be hung to dry in bunches, and the seeds pinched off and rubbed through a sieve once dry.

# Barks

Remember that ringing a tree – removing bark in a ring encircling the trunk – will kill it. However, trees are generally very capable of repairing small patches of missing bark, so taking palm-sized amounts often works well, but do check first that the tree in question looks healthy, and also check those growing locally to it. If any neighbouring trees look unhealthy, or you had noticed that they looked unhealthy earlier in the year when they had leaves, don't take bark from trees in that area as it will weaken them and allow any local diseases to get into the bark and trunk. I generally prefer to prune off small branches and strip the bark from them for medicine-making purposes, but many herbalists have their own preferred methods for this. A paring knife or small bushcraft knife should work well for stripping bark – remember to peel away from yourself in order to avoid cutting your hands. Do be aware that in many countries, including the UK, you cannot legally carry a knife in the open, so if you are foraging for bark, take a bag with you and store your small bushcrafting blade well wrapped and at the bottom of the bag. Alternatively, take some secateurs with you, harvest small branches and bring them home for preparation.

At home, it is time to strip the bark from the branch. I find that a small paring knife works well for this – braced at a 45-degree angle against the twig or branch and pushed firmly away from you, it should take off strips and pieces of bark, including the inner pith, without too much difficulty. Once you have stripped the bark off, it can either be used as it is, or chopped down into much smaller pieces and dried in much the same way as roots, as described above. When dry, store the bark in clean glass jars that have been carefully labelled. Remember when peeling bark to ensure you get as much of the inner pith as possible, as this is usually the part that contains the highest medicinal values.

# Fruit

Many fruits can be gathered when ripe, but some, such as sloes and rosehips, often benefit from freezing overnight as a way to break down the skins and allow their beneficial properties to be released more easily into water or other fluid. This is a useful step if the fruit has been gathered before the first proper frost of the year and is still very hard to the touch. Fruit can be more difficult than other parts of the plant to dry, though some fruits will do very well in a dehydrator.

Hawthorn is usually best gathered from September onwards – you will often find tiny fruit grubs inside the fruit, especially when gathered later on. These are not poisonous and can be picked out of any recipes you've used hawthorn berries in, such as ketchup. Rosehips need to have the irritating seeds and hairs in the centre stripped out before drying, which is a time-consuming job; it is definitely worth at least partially freezing the rosehips first to make it easier to chop them in half. Freshly picked before the first frosts arrive, the skins are so smooth that knives have the bad habit of sliding off, which is how accidents can happen. Many people prefer to just freeze the rosehips whole and use them as needed, but small quantities of rosehips can be prepared, chopped and dried for adding to teas and infusions.

# Medicine making

Roots, bark and seeds need to be bashed up in a mortar and pestle before using them. Seeds should break down fairly well this way – they don't need to be powdered to extract properly, merely thoroughly bruised. For both dried and fresh roots and seeds, a good pounding with a mortar and pestle begins to break down their tough outer layers and will therefore allow better access of water, alcohol or oil during medicine making, which will result in a more effective preparation. Roots and bark are easier to work with when pounded thoroughly using a good heavy mortar and pestle, which will help them extract more efficiently into water. My preferred technique for bashing up seeds is to partially cover the mortar with one hand and give the seeds good, firm taps with the pestle, used through the space left open between hand and mortar. This reduces the likelihood of the seeds ricocheting around the kitchen. Once the seeds have been roughly broken down, you can work the pestle in circles around the mortar, grinding the seeds more firmly against the sides.

Decoctions are the preferred water-extraction method for tougher plant parts, such as seeds, roots and bark, and there are two different methods you can use. Short decoctions can be made by allowing 1 tbsp of the chopped roots to 570 ml (20 fl oz) of water, and then simmering the lot on a moderate heat until the liquid quantity has reduced by about half. Long decoctions are simmered for several hours, with equivalent amounts of herbs and water, but the water level is topped up from time to time to really give the water time to get the best out of the roots. This process can be fascinating to watch as an almost oily layer forms on top of the liquid over a period of hours. Short decoctions can last up to three days when stored in a fridge, and are taken in approximately half-cup (120 ml) doses, while long decoctions can last months when kept in the fridge, and are taken in 1 tbsp (15 ml) doses.

Tinctures need to be made using the strongest alcohol you can get, and I tend to prefer to let them steep for twice as long as leafy tinctures to really allow them to extract properly into the alcohol. If you are using dried roots or seeds, leave for at least four weeks before straining out the spent herbs, and use at least 35% proof alcohol, if at all possible. You can use vodka, brandy, gin, rum or any kind of alcohol you prefer, but remember that tinctures are made to act as medicines – they are taken in small doses.

If you choose to buy a tincture, this will be specified as a ratio followed by a percentage, such as 1:3 40%. Here, the ratio signifies that 3 ml of liquid contains 1 g of the herb, and 40% indicates the percentage of alcohol in the liquid.

This is only a very brief introduction to medicine making with roots, seeds, barks and fruits – further hints and tips will be included with the herbs covered in this book, as needed.

## *Autumn and winter herbs for the medicine garden*

There is a range of herbs that make great additions to the medicine garden and are suitable for gathering in the late summer, autumn and winter. Here is a very brief, but by no means exhaustive, list – why not grow a few of these beauties yourself?

**Angelica** (*Angelica archangelica*) would have to be first on the list. This beautiful and statuesque plant gives warming medicine for the stomach and circulation and produces masses of bright-green leaves, huge flower heads of pale-green flowers in its second year of growth, and plentiful amounts of seeds in the autumn. Remember to plant some of those seeds straight from the flower head if you would like to propagate your plant.

**Blue flag** (*Iris versicolor*) is a water-loving plant and makes a beautiful display in a water garden – but if you don't have a pond or an aquatic environment for it, why not grow it in a large pot instead? Don't drill any holes in the bottom of the pot, but keep the plant well watered and it will reward you all summer with masses of beautiful leaves and a flowering season of purple flowers followed by fascinating seed heads.

**Calamus** (*Acorus calamus*) root gives valuable medicine as well, and can be planted alongside blue flag plants if you like, although they can sometimes be drowned out by them. If you are worried that your calamus root may not survive the battle with the blue flag, give it its own separate water pot and it will reward you with masses of fragrant roots.

**Chicory** (*Chicorium intybus*) gives beautiful blue flowers all summer, followed by bitter, but tasty and nourishing roots in the autumn. If you'd like to make your own chicory coffee, you might want to consider growing a whole patch of these handsome plants.

**Cramp bark** (*Viburnum opulus*) makes a beautiful hedge and a very lovely, showy plant in the garden as well, with masses of snowy flowers in the spring leading to autumnal shows of red and purple foliage punctuated with semi-translucent, glossy red berries much beloved by birds.

**Marshmallow** (*Althaea officinalis*) flowers all summer, and the flowers and leaves can be gathered then for medicine making. The root of this perennial can be dug up in the autumn for its soothing properties.

**Sweet cicely** (*Myrrhis odorata*) produces filmy, fern-like foliage all summer, with a flowering season of delicate white blooms in May. Later in the summer and autumn, substantial seed heads are produced, which start out green and turn a glossy black over time. Both these and the roots make great food and equally good medicine.

Last, but not least, would have to be **yarrow** (*Achillea millefolium*). There are several brightly coloured cultivars of this wonderful medicinal plant, but for the useful sorts, go for the traditional variety (check the Latin name, to be sure that is what you've got). Plant it in a place that gives it not particularly good soil, and you should get plenty of aromatic flowers from late summer through most of autumn.

# Angelica
## *Angelica archangelica / Archangelica officinalis*

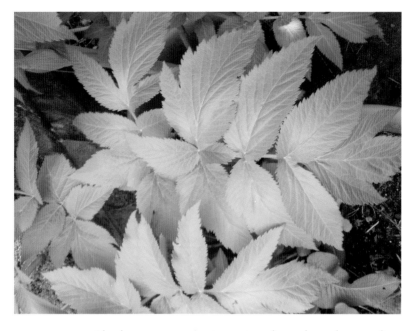

*Also known as:*  masterwort, archangel, garden angelica,
the angel's herb, bellyache root, root of the Holy Ghost,
herba angelica (angel's plant)

**Family**  Apiaceae.

**Habitat and description**  Angelica is a biennial that grows
to a height of 2.5 m (8 ft) or more, dwarfing all other
herbs in the herb garden given half a chance. The leaves
are bright, spring green, and large and lobed in shape, divid-
ing into smaller sections. They smell aromatic and pungent,
with a strong hint of celery, and make a rather tasty tea.
The stem is thick and hollow, with ridges running around it,

and the younger stems have been used for quite some time to make brilliant-green candied angelica for cake decorating. The flowers are white and palest green, grow in wide umbels, and appear during July and August of the plant's second year of growth, vigorous and beautiful expressions of the plant's vitality.

The root, when used in medicine, is gathered at the end of the first year, in late autumn when the energy of the plant has retreated back into the ground. The plant grows readily in damp soil, particularly loving to grow near running water, and in shady spots, and can be propagated by seed or by root division. If you would like to grow it from seed, it needs to be done using seed freshly gathered from the plant and planted straight back into the earth, as it is notoriously tricky to cultivate from stored seed.

**Where to find it**    Angelica grows wild in parts of Europe and Scandinavia, and is easily cultivated in most temperate regions of the world. It can also be found in North America.

**Parts used**    Leaves, roots and seeds.

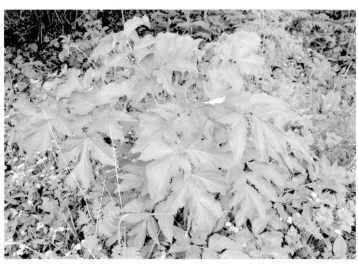

**When to gather**    The root at the end of the first year; seeds after flowering; leaves in spring and summer.

**Medicines to make**    Infused oils, vinegars, wines, candied peel, candied seeds, seeds stored for chewing. You can also make a tincture of the root, and a tea of the leaves for easing dyspepsia and toning a digestive system that is prone to dampness and inefficiency.

**Constituents**    Volatile oil (especially the root and seeds), which contains monoterpenes such as limonene; coumarins, especially furanocoumarin glycosides, as well as angelicin, umbelliferone, psoralen (responsible for photosensitivity in some people) and bergapten; and miscellaneous sugars, plant acids and flavonoids, such as archangelenone and sterols.

**Planetary influence**    The sun.

**Associated deities and heroes**    Michael, Sun Gods such as Helios, Lugh, Apollo, Freyr and Ra; also associated with Venus. It could, by extension, also be associated with Sun Goddesses, although these are fewer in number than their male counterparts. Some Sun Goddesses include Sunna / Sol and Amaterasu.

**Festival**    Winter Solstice, Imbolc, Summer Solstice. (Different folk have different opinions on the festival associated with this herb. Personally, I think associating it with the Summer Solstice makes most sense in terms of the plant and its qualities; however, I can see the logic of associating it with the Winter Solstice and Imbolc as well, in terms of the pagan myth of the rebirth of the sun that occurs annually at this time of year.) Ultimately, it is entirely up to the reader which of these festivals they feel most suits the plant.

**Constitution**    Warm and dry. Angelica is ruled by the element of Fire (unsurprisingly, given its planetary influence!).

**Actions and indications**    Our old friend Culpeper wrote that angelica was used to build immunity and resistance against the plague and other epidemical diseases. Fortunately for us these days, the plague is less of a problem, though the immune-boosting properties can still come in handy! The root and stalk can be used to warm a cold stomach, and can also be used in general for any cold, airy diseases of the body. Culpeper also reckons that it is used to bring on periods, and to treat strangury and colic. Externally, he says, it can be used to treat ulcers, bites, gout and sciatica.

These days angelica is used as a smooth-muscle relaxant and carminative, making it great for relieving wind, bloating and colic. It is expectorant and antispasmodic, so can be used to relieve congested coughs, and is a gentle digestive tonic. The herb contains coumarin, which in this case has a reputation as a cancer inhibitor. It has been previously used as a tonic for those in the later stages of life, as it boosts and supports the circulation and is a warming tonic to the digestion. I've used it to good effect for wind caused by impaired-digestion and for bloating, constipation and headaches that do not respond to conventional painkillers, in which respect it is somewhat similar to blue flag and could be combined with it to make an effective digestive medicine.

The plant has a bitter principle but is usually used as an aromatic tonic; the volatile oil has carminative qualities, with similar actions to that of wormwood (*Artemisia absinthium*), though considerably less bitter. An oil made of the leaves can be used externally to treat rheumatism and arthritis.

The leaves can be used as a diaphoretic, to help the body break out in a sweat and lower the temperature in the case of fevers and influenza. It can also be taken to help the body recover after illness as it is warming and strengthening.

As it is warming and stimulating to the circulation, it can be used to relieve a variety of issues relating to blood and the circulatory system, including anaemia, Raynaud's disease and peripheral vascular disease. As a herb with an affinity for the chest, it can be used as part of treatment plans for a wide variety of respiratory issues including coughs, catarrh, bronchitis, asthma and related problems. Its aromatic content also makes it handy for treating digestive issues ranging from nervous dyspepsia to colic and lack of appetite.

Externally, the oil or a poultice of the leaves can be used to treat pleurisy and bronchitis, or the leaves can be steeped in alcohol to make a warming liniment for arthritis and rheumatism. As part of a cream, angelica can be used to heal and soothe radiation damage to the skin.

The root also has an affinity for the liver, helping the production of bile and improving the metabolism of oils. The whole plant can be used to relieve headaches, chills, aches and pains, neuralgia and myalgia, as it warms and supports the system.

For women, the plant can be helpful as well, easing PMS and depression and bringing on the menses, though it should be avoided if pregnancy is suspected or already present.

**Folklore**     Unsurprisingly enough given the name of the plant, it is commonly believed that the plant was put here by assorted different angels – a fact that Culpeper makes a number of amusing and rather pithy comments about, relating to the age-old tradition of naming plants after various saints, angels and holy figures. In Culpeper's opinion, the physicians of his age were copying the ancient tradition but for totally the wrong reasons!

There is an old tradition in Eastern Europe of gathering the flower stems of wild plants, then carrying them back into the village and offering them for sale while chanting an ancient song or verse in unintelligible words that are not even understood by the people singing them. It's entirely possible that this tradition is a carryover from an ancient pagan custom. The words and tune of the song are learned in early childhood, so it is feasible that the words used to make sense but have become distorted over the generations. There is an old legend stating that the herb was revealed as a plague cure by an angel appearing in a dream. The name is also explained by the fact that it apparently flowers on the day of Michael the Archangel – May 8th – making it a herb of this particular angel. It's possible that this connection explains the plant's long and venerable history of use to ward off witches and evil spirits.

**Dose**    Tincture dosage is 1–3 ml of 1:3 strength tincture in 35% alcohol for the root, or 5 ml of the leaf tincture. Cold infusion or decoction of the herb should be 6–12 g per cup of water.

**Contraindications**    Do not use during pregnancy, as the herb is an emmenagogue. Some consider that the herb should not be used by diabetics because of the high sugar content of the plant. Use of the herb can cause photosensitivity in some individuals. This herb would not suit people with excessively hot constitutions. Use with caution in cases of hyperacidity or peptic ulceration, or duodenitis and gastro-oesophageal reflux, as this herb is very warming and will not suit these issues. Seek medical advice before using if you are already taking warfarin or another blood thinner.

# Angelica recipes

## Herbal bitters

**Ingredients**
- » vodka or brandy
- » an assortment of digestive herbs, such as: dandelion root, angelica seeds or root, fennel, orange or lemon peel, lavender, chamomile etc.

**Instructions**    This is very simple indeed to make. Just add 5 g of each herb you would like to include to a Kilner jar, and then cover with vodka until there is a centimetre or so on top of the herbs. Tighten the lid and leave the concoction for two weeks, shaking it up daily. Take a few drops before or after a meal to stimulate the digestion. You can use orange peel, lavender, fennel and dill or vanilla to flavour the bitters, and you can even sweeten them with a tiny bit of honey if you want, but remember that the bitter kick still has to come through in order to be effective on the digestion, as by stimulating the vagus nerve in the mouth, bitters encourage the digestion to produce more digestive enzymes. Adding dandelion root or even filter coffee can also improve the bitter effects as well as stimulating the bowels in cases of constipation.

## Angelica leaf balm for rheumatism and arthritis

**Ingredients**
- » plenty of fresh angelica leaves picked on a dry day
- » organic seed or vegetable oil
- » beeswax
- » juniper essential oil

**Instructions**    Finely chop the clean, dry leaves and pile them into a double boiler, covering them with the oil and infusing the whole lot on a moderate heat for at least half an hour. Strain out the first batch of leaves and add a second batch to get a stronger oil, repeating the process. When the oil is as strong as you wish it to be, add 12 g of beeswax per 100 ml (3½ fl oz) of oil and return the lot to the double boiler, heating and stirring until the beeswax has melted. Add 5 drops of juniper essential oil, and stir the balm briefly to disperse the scent thoroughly. Pour the resulting balm into jars, putting the lid on once cool and labelling carefully with the name and date of the preparation. Rub into sore joints caused by rheumatism and arthritis. This balm is also lovely used on sore muscles post-training.

## Angelica digestive tonic

**Ingredients**
- » angelica leaves, stems, seeds and root
- » vodka or brandy

**Instructions**    This is a recipe that needs to be made slowly, through the year, and you will probably need two plants for it. Gather the leaves and stems in the spring, clean and chop them, and pile them into a Kilner jar, covering them with the alcohol. Leave them to steep in a cool, dark cupboard, shaking regularly. The seeds can be gathered in late summer, crushed in a mortar and pestle, and then added to the jar. In the autumn, add some fresh root from a first-year plant, dug up in October or November. Scrub the root thoroughly, chop it finely, and add it to the concoction, adding more alcohol if needed. Steep the whole lot for another month once the last ingredient has been added, then strain out the herbs and pour the liquid into a bottle. To use, decant into a small dropper bottle and label it with the name and dosage, and take 10 drops three times a day for digestive issues. This can be taken as it is, or it can be added to a small glass of water.

# Apple / crab apple
## Malus pumila / Malus sylvestris

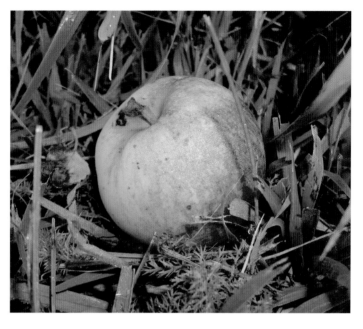

*Also known as:* fruit of the Underworld, scrab, bittersgall, gribble, grindstone apple, scrogg, sour grapes, wilding-tree, fruit of the gods, silver branch, the silver bough, tree of love

**Family**   Rosaceae. A common synonym for the apple (*Malus pumila*) is *Pyrus malus.*

**Habitat and description**   The apple and crab apple are very similar in terms of habitat and description. The crab apple (*Malus sylvestris*) is an attractive tree, growing to a height of some 9 m (30 ft), with a trunk girth of up to 3 m (10 ft). It can often be found growing in hedgerows and copses, and with age develops some amazing twisted, contorted shapes like the traditional fairy-tale witch. The leaves are roughly oval in shape, and the tree bears many pale pink and cream, fragrant flowers in spring. The apples are smaller, harder versions of our domestic apples and are usually too tart to eat straight from the bough. They do, however, make wonderful jelly and preserves and were often used in punches and alcoholic beverages.

When I was a child, we had a venerable old crab apple growing in our garden, which seemed to have a very kindly, benevolent feel to it, although the shape of the tree itself was very contorted and twisted after many years of growth. The bark was deeply fissured and a deep greyish brown in colour, and every autumn it produced a heavy crop of crab apples, most of which ended up scattered around on the grass with an abundance of wasps feeding on them.

Apple trees of all kinds can be found growing along

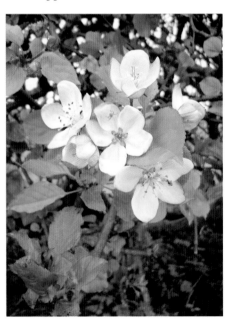

the sides of roads, in woodland, wasteland, meadows, old orchards, gardens . . . the list is endless.

**Where to find it**   Apples can be found growing in gardens, hedgerows and woodlands in most temperate regions of the world, including Europe, North America and parts of Scandinavia.

**Parts used**   Bark, fruit (remember the old saying: "an apple a day keeps the doctor away"?).

**When to gather**   Late summer and autumn.

**Medicines to make**   Infusions and vinegars; fruit as a food; baked-apple poultices.

**Constituents**   The apple fruit contains iron, malic acid and pectin, as well as sugars, fruit acids, vitamins A, B1 and C and minerals. These useful constituents live just under the apple skin, meaning that to get the full value of the fruit it should be eaten whole, not peeled; this is the main reason why unpasteurised cider vinegar is so full of medicinal properties. The bark of the apple tree contains quercetin and is bitter. The seeds contain cyanide and amygdaline and are poisonous if eaten in large quantities.

**Planetary influence**   Venus.

**Associated deities and heroes**   Aphrodite, King Arthur, Athene, Cerridwen, Diana, Eve, Flora, Godiva, Grannos, Herakles, Hermes, The Hesperides, Iduna, Mabon, Modron, Olwen, Titaea, The Triple Goddess, Venus, Helen of Troy, Astarte, Ashtoreth, Ishtar, Nemesis, Eurystheus, Gwen, Arwen, Shekinah, Atlas, Paris and Cupid – quite a list! Apples feature in a plethora of old myths, legends and folktales.

**Festival**   Mabon, the Autumn Equinox.

**Constitution**   Cool and moist – the fruit of the crab apple is very sour in taste.

**Actions and indications**   It is predominantly cultivated apple that is used for medicine making these days, as it provides a sweeter remedy that is easier to work with. Crab apples tend to be a lot smaller, tarter and harder, and while they can still be used, they can have a much sharper flavour. The apple is a digestive stimulant, lowers cholesterol levels, and is laxative and nutritive, so basically it has quite a link with the digestive system in general, especially in unpasteurised vinegar form.

The fruit of the cultivated apple can be made into a useful and tasty tea for fevers, and baked apples have traditionally been used in poultices to treat sore throats, fever and inflammation. Apples can be used to clear blood toxins and are good for the teeth and gums. In the past the fresh fruit has been recommended for constipation, rheumatism, high cholesterol, indigestion and diarrhoea. The dried peel can be made into a tea for rheumatism, perhaps pointing towards a general anti-inflammatory action of the fruit. This is interesting in light of the school of thinking that indicates that most ill health develops from inflammation of some part of the body – therefore, the old saying "an apple a day keeps the doctor away" would make a great deal of sense!

The fruit can be used in the control of hypoglycaemia, possibly due to its high pectin content, which is also responsible for its anti-cholesterol properties. Eating an apple regularly can also guard the body against heart disease and cancer. The flowers and leaves can be combined into a tea to ward off hayfever.

I think it is important to talk a bit more about apple cider vinegar here, in particular the unpasteurised version. This delightful stuff has a reputation these days for helping relieve a wide variety of health issues, including improving hearing, fighting viruses, improving and boosting the immune system, relieving fatigue, speeding up the metabolism and thereby assisting in weight loss, relieving constipation and keeping the bowels regular. There has also been some mention recently of it being used to improve cancer survival rates by a fairly dramatic amount. All in all, handy to have as a regular part of your diet!

**Folklore**    Traditionally, unicorns live underneath apple trees. There is a huge body of folklore about the apple, ranging from magical silver branches in Irish lore to the magical tree of the Hesperides in Greek myths and legends.

The apple tree already had a long association with the Summerlands when it became linked to the fabled Isle of Avalon, or Isle of Apples, the final resting place of the great King Arthur, taken there by the nine Morgans after his fateful death at the great battle of Camlann. Of course, this was not the first mention of the sacred apple in Celtic and British myths and legends – the tree is also mentioned several times in the Celtic tales of the Mabinogion, perhaps most notably at the beginning of the Voyage of King Bran the Blessed, who, when he fell asleep outside the gates of his citadel one morning as the result of ethereal music that only he could hear, was greeted on awakening with the sight of a beautiful silver branch laden with apples and white blossom. He took the branch back into his hall, and when he did, an ethereal woman appeared in the centre of the room and sang a haunting, fey song about the Otherworld. When the song finished, she vanished, taking the magical silver branch with her. Of course, this song lit a fire in the soul of King Bran, and nothing would please him then but to set sail on a long search for the Otherworld, also marking the beginning of a saga of many adventures, losses and hard-won wisdom. This is only one of many legends and myths linking the apple with both the Gods and the Otherworld – Idunn, one of the Norse Goddesses, possessed the Apples of Immortality which the

Norse Gods ate on a regular basis to keep them forever young and immortal.

Over the other side of the world, the apple was the message that brought about the downfall of Troy as young Paris was given an apple to present to the Goddess he thought fairest. He chose Aphrodite, who gave him Helen as a reward. The garden of the Hesperides had a mythical apple tree, the apples from which Hercules was sent to steal. These are only a few of the legends surrounding the humble apple – there are many, many more.

**Dose**    Fruit – as much as you like, though large doses will give you diarrhoea and a bad stomach. Bark and leaf – no more than 15 drops per day of a weak tincture; for a weak tincture, go for 1:10 30% proof or thereabouts.

**Contraindications**    Care should be taken when using the bark or leaf medicinally as they contain cyanogenic glycosides that can be fatally toxic in large doses.

# Apple recipes

## Apple cider vinegar

**Ingredients / equipment**
   » windfall apples – bruised and battered works just fine, but nothing too mouldy or insect-eaten. Alternatively, use the peel, core and bruised bits from apples you will be cooking with – either is fine.
   » water
   » a large bucket with a lid, or something similar
   » a corner in an airing cupboard, or somewhere warm and dry

**Instructions**    Roughly chop or shred the apples or the apple peel and core – don't go too mad with this, as I find it makes perfectly good vinegar even if the pieces are still rather large! Pack it all into a large bucket with a lid, pour over enough water to cover the apples, then pop the lid on. Put the bucket into the airing cupboard or somewhere similar, and stir it every couple of days. After a few days there will be the distinct smell of apples in the area, and a couple of days after that it will smell as though the apples are fermenting. Leave the apples in for as long as you like, until the vinegar is as strong as you want it to be, then strain out the apples. Leave the sediment in – this is the vinegar mother, the bit that is particularly good for you.

This vinegar makes a lovely vehicle for herbs, so you can use it to make herbal honegars – basically chopped herbs, vinegar and honey – as well as using it for a variety of other recipes. I find 1 tbsp (15 ml) of vinegar in a cup of warm water with a large pinch of cinnamon and a dollop of honey is a lovely drink, tasting rather like autumn in a cup. It is also superb for relieving simple diarrhoea. Topically, dilute the vinegar with an equal amount of aromatic water, such as rose water, to make an astringent skin treatment that restores the pH of skin and relieves redness and acne. You can make aromatic waters at home if you have an alembic and access to a *lot* of flowers, but it's easier just to buy them. They are a by-product of the essential oil industry, and a good source for them is places that sell aromatherapy supplies or products for making bath and body treatments.

## Apple cider vinegar – a second method

### Ingredients
- » freshly pressed apple juice – plenty of it
- » vinegar mother from unpasteurised cider vinegar

**Instructions**    This is really simple to make – just pour the apple juice into a demijohn and allow it to ferment, and then to turn to vinegar. Don't filter out any of the sediment at the bottom – this is the mother, the most valuable part of the vinegar. You can add some of the mother from unpasteurised cider vinegar if you have any spare – I keep the bottom few centimetres from old batches for this purpose, as it can be used to kick-start new batches of vinegar.

## Tonic vinegars made with cider vinegar

**Ingredients**
  » fresh or dried herbs, such as peppermint and meadowsweet (for digestive upsets) or lemon balm and chamomile (for stress)
  » unpasteurised cider vinegar

**Instructions**    Tonic vinegars are very simple to make. Choose what sort of action you would like for your tonic vinegar to have, and gather the herbs accordingly. If you are using fresh herbs, allow 1 heaped tablespoon of each kind of herb per 570 ml of vinegar, up to 10 heaped tablespoons. If you are using dry herbs, level tablespoons should work just as well. Pile the herbs and unpasteurised cider vinegar into a jar and let the whole lot infuse for at least a fortnight, then filter the resulting concoction and bottle it. To take the infused vinegar, just add 1 tbsp (15 ml) to 570 ml (20 fl oz) of cool water once a day and sip it. Try to avoid pouring boiling water onto the vinegar if possible, as this destroys the vinegar mother. Herb-infused cider vinegars can also be used as skin washes and toners, and as cleaning agents around the house. They also make delicious salad dressings and dips, and are very tasty added to houmous instead of lemon juice.

## Apple and rosehip pudding

**Ingredients**
  » cooking apples
  » rosehip syrup (see Rose recipes)
  » cinnamon
  » mixed fruit
  » slivered almonds or chopped hazelnuts
  » organic rolled oats – at least 4 heaped tablespoons
  » organic butter or coconut oil
  » maple syrup or local honey
  » cream or ice cream to serve

**Instructions**   Peel and core the apples, slice them roughly, and pile them into an oven-proof dish, then scatter over a good handful of the mixed fruit and the nuts. Sprinkle a liberal amount of cinnamon over the top of the fruit, then pour over a steady trickle of rosehip syrup – you are aiming to moisten the fruit, not drench it, as the apples will cook down and release their own juices.

In a separate pan, add 50 g (1¾ oz) of butter or coconut oil and warm it through until it melts, then add the maple syrup or honey. Once the two are mixed thoroughly, add the oats and stir them in thoroughly until they are coated with the sticky mixture. You can either top the fruit with this immediately or, if you think the oats are a bit too sticky, add a few more oats to soak up the mixture. Sprinkle the oat mix over the top of the fruit, and put the whole thing in the oven at around 170°C for 15 minutes, until the fruit is bubbling, the apples have broken down, and the oats are golden brown. Serve hot, with cream or ice cream.

# Blue flag
## *Iris versicolor*

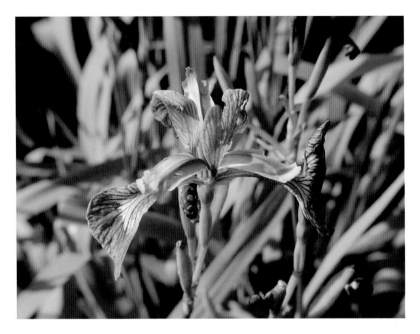

*Also known as:*   water flag, purple iris, liver lily, fleur-de-lys

**Family**   Iridaceae.

**Habitat and description**   A water-loving plant, blue flag thrives in pond margins and the edges of rivers and streams, where it throws up sword-shaped leaves in profusion, forming elegant fans, followed in the summer by tall, cylindrical stalks featuring the characteristic pale-blue and yellow flowers, which last for a couple of days and are absolutely beautiful to behold. Each flower features three sets of petals – the first three curve gently downwards; the second three arch out horizontally; and the final set arch skywards, with yellow colouring and pronounced deep-indigo veins on the lower petals. Later on, seed heads are produced, each slowly peeling open to reveal a plethora of shiny, round seeds, which are a rich chestnut in colour. Blue flag grows very happily in pots as long as it is well watered, making the harvesting of the roots somewhat easier. It also grows perfectly well as a garden plant, though I find it thrives best in good, damp soil. The plant grows up to 75 cm (30 in.) tall and, given enough space and plenty of water, will form huge mats of growth. The roots grow from creeping rhizomes that allow the plant to spread out.

**Where to find it**   Canada, Eastern USA, UK and Ireland.

**Parts used**   Roots and rhizomes.

**When to gather**   Late autumn and early winter, early spring.

**Medicines to make**   Tinctures and elixirs, decoctions, vinegars, dried root.

**Constituents**   Triterpenoid acids including salicylic acid; volatile oils, tannins, sterols and resins; Iridin / Irisin, which is the predominant liver active component.

**Planetary influence**   Moon.

**Associated deities and heroes**   Iris, the rainbow Goddess; Juno.

**Festival**   None known at present.

**Constitution**   Warm and dry.

**Actions and indications**   Blue flag has a particular affinity with the digestive tract, perhaps most especially the liver, making it ideal for hepatic disorders such as chronic hepatitis, indigestion, pancreatic and splenic enlargement and insufficiency, fatty liver, constipation, and bilious headache due to upset stomach function. It can also be used to relieve jaundice due to its tonic effect on liver function. It is an irritant bitter, which improves and increases secretions and corrects faulty digestion, but it needs to be used in small doses only, as larger doses can cause nausea. It combines well with other digestive medicines such as dandelion root, meadowsweet leaf, and mucous membrane tonics like plantain (*Plantago lanceolata* or *P. major*). One particular symptom pattern it works well with is constipation combined with wind causing griping pains, and with a frontal headache that tends to be a cluster, moving from one side to the other and not responding well to conventional painkillers. Blue flag combined with peppermint and fennel as drop doses can be really effective, as can blue flag combined with angelica.

As a diuretic, blue flag can be used to improve overall kidney health as well as to act as a useful medicine for the relief of kidney infections, when combined with soothing herbs such as corn silk and couch grass.

Blood sugar issues can be improved by the use of blue flag, as its stimulant effects on the liver encourage better management and storage of blood sugars after eating. It combines well with cinnamon for this purpose.

As a vasotonic alterative, it can also be used to alleviate

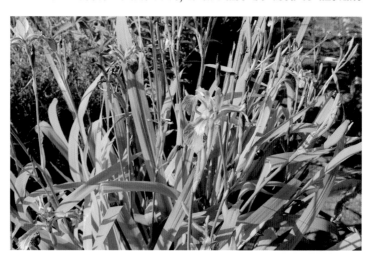

some skin diseases, including acne, as part of a lymphatic mixture with cleavers. It can be of benefit in cases of eczema and psoriasis as well, by encouraging the outward movement of heat, which, when trapped in the liver and causing inflammation and reduced liver function, can often worsen these skin issues. Add cleavers topically as well if you are treating psoriasis, and be aware of the healing crisis that treating these two ailments can often precipitate, which causes the issue to get worse to begin with before it gets better. I find this usually happens because the heat stored in the liver has to go somewhere and is often released through the skin, worsening the complaint before things begin to settle down.

The vasotonic alterative effect can also be helpful with rheumatic complaints, and blue flag can be combined with herbs suited to the treatment of rheumatism and arthritis, as well as other herbs that will encourage better flow of blood and elimination of waste from the system.

Lastly, the herb has a reputation for being handy in the case of enlarged thyroid, where it can be used to moderate sudden changes, such as those brought on by high levels of stress. Combine it with adaptogens and nervines for this purpose – skullcap is a good one to bear in mind. The herb also moderates sudden mood swings, such as those caused by liver distress.

**Folklore**   Named for the Goddess of rainbows, Iris, due to the range of colour in the petals, blue flag (*Iris versicolor*) also has links with Juno, queen of the Greek gods, as well as having seen use in ancient Egypt, where it was used to adorn the Sphinx and the sceptres of their kings. Orris, another member of the Iris family, has famously been used for hundreds of years in perfumery and is also a valuable ingredient in a range of other items, including scented beads, potpourri and fragrant pillows, where it acts as a fixative as well as providing a scent of its own.

Blue flag has a long history of use by the Native American tribes and was often found growing near their villages.

**Dose**    No more than 6 ml of the tincture per day, though other sources recommend drop doses only – I use approximately 1 tbsp (15 ml) in a week's prescription to good effect, though drop doses for digestive issues should certainly be very effective. Higher doses than this will cause nausea and potentially vomiting.

**Contraindications**    Can cause nausea. Avoid during pregnancy.

# Blue flag recipes

## Tonic for poor digestion

**Ingredients**
  » fresh blue flag root
  » fresh meadowsweet leaves
  » fresh dandelion root
  » fresh mint leaves
  » vodka

**Instructions**    Carefully wash the blue flag root and then grate it thoroughly. Check over the rest of the herbs you want to include and finely chop them using a mezzaluna or food processor, then pile the lot into a Kilner jar. Ideally you want roughly equal parts of each herb. The vodka or other alcohol used needs to be as strong as you can manage, in order to ensure your tonic blend will keep for longer – alcohol diluted below 25% proof has a much shorter keeping time, and fresh herbs contain a high quantity of water that will dilute the alcohol by a surprising amount. If you are worried about the alcohol not keeping long enough, let the herbs wilt overnight before you chop and use them, just to allow a little of the liquid content to evaporate. Once the herbs are chopped and packed into a jar, pour over enough vodka to cover the herbs, with an extra couple of centimetres on top, and let the whole thing steep for at least a week, two if possible, shaking it all up regularly. Once you are happy with how strong the tonic blend is, filter it off, and bottle it. Pour some of the tonic into a dropper bottle and label it, then take 5 drops half an hour before meals to encourage better, more comfortable digestion and to act as a tonic to the stomach and liver.

## Blood sugar tonic

**Ingredients**
- » fresh or dried blue flag root
- » dandelion root
- » cinnamon
- » vodka or brandy (if making the tincture)
- » 1.2 l (40 fl oz) of filtered or spring water (if making the long decoction)

**Instructions**    This tonic can be made as a tincture or a long decoction. To make the tincture, start by scrubbing the blue flag root – if you are using it fresh – and do the same with the dandelion root. Grate or finely chop the roots and pack them into a Kilner jar, then add 1 tbsp of powdered cinnamon, or grind up two cinnamon sticks and pile them in. Cover the herbs with the alcohol, allowing the usual extra couple of centimetres on top, and pop the lid on, leaving the whole mixture to infuse for at least a fortnight. If you use dried roots, you will need to leave it for at least twice that amount of time to allow the alcohol to extract the medicinal properties from the dried herbs and spices as fully as possible. The tincture dosage is ½ tsp (2.5 ml) twice a day.

Alternatively, you can make a long decoction of the roots. Pile the dried roots into a saucepan or slow cooker, add 1 tsp, heaped, of ground cinnamon, then add 1.2 l (40 fl oz) of filtered or spring water. Bring to a steady simmer and allow to simmer for at least two hours, four if possible. If you are making this recipe on the hob, keep topping up with water as the liquid evaporates. Eventually you should find you have about 570 ml (20 fl oz) of liquid left, which may be thicker and even slightly oily on the surface. Filter off the finished long decoction, compost the spent herbs, and then bottle the liquid. Once it is cool, store it in the fridge or in a cool cupboard, and take about 2 tsp (10 ml) before each meal, adjusting the dosage as needed. You'll know if you have had too much, as it will give you a slightly funny stomach, in which case reduce the dose. This method can also be used for the digestive tonic recipe. Make sure you remember to label the bottle carefully with the ingredients, date and dosage.

## Blue flag tincture

**Ingredients**
  » plenty of fresh or dried blue flag root
  » alcohol of your choice

**Instructions**   Scrub and finely chop or grate the roots, then pile them into a Kilner jar and cover them with plenty of the alcohol, allowing an extra couple of centimetres on top. Leave it to steep for at least two weeks, longer if you are using dried roots, then filter off the alcohol and store it. Use small amounts – ½ tsp (2.5 ml) twice a day is usually plenty.

# Burdock
## *Arctium lappa*

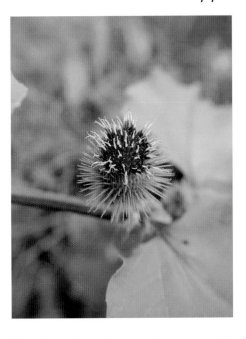

*Also known as:*   appa, fox's clote, thorny burr, beggar's buttons, cockle buttons, love leaves, philanthropium, prosopium personata, happy major, clot-bur, bardana, burrseed, cockleburr, great burdock, hardock, hurrburr, sweethearts, cuckoo button, bardona, grass burdock, hareburr, cuckold buttons, donkeys, eddick, flapper-bags, gypsy comb, kisses, loppy major, pig's rhubarb, sticky jacks, touch-me-not, tuzzy-muzzy, wild rhubarb, burr-top

**Family**   Asteraceae.

**Habitat and description**   Burdock is a tall, stately biennial, growing to approximately 1.5 m (5 ft) tall, with large, roughly oval, ruffle-edged leaves and a tall central stem, bearing lots of small, bristly seed heads, which follow tufted purple flowers that have a thistle-like appearance. The seeds tend to stick to anything that brushes past them, hence many of the folk names for the plant. The root is harvested in the first autumn or second spring (when the tonic effect is apparently more pronounced) and takes a great deal of digging to unearth, as it burrows deep. If you want to gather burdock, set aside a goodly amount of time for the digging of it – this is a plant that makes you work for your medicine! The leaves have a pleasant aromatic scent, with dark-green upper leaves and pale silvery-grey undersides. The young plant grows close to the ground, around a basal rosette of leaves. The young leaves are roughly heart-shaped and tend to be very aromatic if you give them a good rub – a delightful surprise! The roots, once unearthed, are gnarly on the outside, with a lovely creamy-coloured, juicy centre, and they can grow up to a metre (3¼ ft)

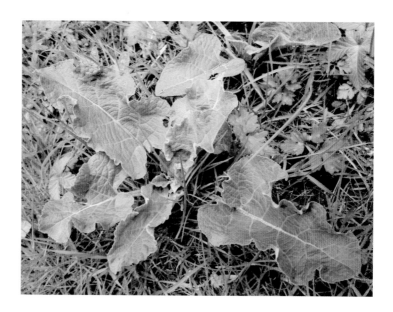

deep – it is difficult to dig the whole thing up, and even the smallest piece of root left in the ground provides enough for the plant to grow back from.

**Where to find it**   Burdock is found in most temperate regions of the world, from Scandinavia to North America, Asia and Europe.

**Parts used**   Root, seeds, leaves.

**When to gather**   Autumn for the root and seeds, summer for the leaves.

**Medicines to make**   Tinctures and vinegars, syrups, infused oils; cooked as food.

**Constituents**   As with most herbs, burdock contains quite a list of constituents, including lignans such as arctigenin and its glycoside, polyacetylenes in the root, sesquiterpenes in the leaves, and up to 50% inulin in the roots, which is better extracted from the fresh plant – drying tends to denature it. The plant also contains assorted organic acids, fatty acids and phenolic acids, including isovaleric and caffeic acid. Trace minerals such as iron, sulphur and B-vitamins as well as mucilage are also present, as well as vitamin C, magnesium, calcium, chromium, phosphorus and potassium.

**Planetary influence**   Venus.

**Associated deities and heroes**   Blodeuwedd, plus assorted water deities due to its affinity with the movement of internal waters; goddesses of the Underworld, such as Hel, Hecate and Cerridwen – anyone trying to dig the root will soon understand why the plant has this link.

**Festival**   I tend to associate this plant with Samhain, but do draw your own conclusions on this.

**Constitution**   Cool and moist.

**Actions and indications**   Burdock is primarily known as a blood cleanser and alterative. It can be used to treat acne and related skin conditions as well as problems such as psoriasis and eczema. Being ruled by Venus, it has a strong affinity with the blood and lymph and stimulates the movement of lymph around the body, causing a cleansing effect that can sometimes worsen a problem before it improves. Burdock root is best given as a low-dosage tonic over longer periods of time to gently stimulate and move the lymph and encourage the body to self-regulate.

The root is cooked and eaten as a root vegetable in Japan, Hawaii and New Zealand, often part-boiled and then cooked in sauce. Burdock is often particularly well suited to encouraging cells to get rid of their waste materials, handy in systems that have become slow and sluggish and bogged down. It combines very well with red clover or dock root, as well as with dandelion root as a traditional detoxifying drink that is far removed from the additive-laden concoctions available in the supermarkets these days. It is also a fantastic blood tonic and has antibiotic and adaptogenic effects, helping us to better cope with stress.

Burdock has been used for many years as a nutritive tonic and deep healer. One of its constituents, arctigenin, can be used in the treatment of cancerous growths and to inhibit tumour development. It has been used to treat the side-effects of chemotherapy and to boost the system to allow it to better fight off cancer, as it is a good immune strengthener. It has also been used alongside other herbs to treat chronic fatigue and autoimmune diseases.

Another of its main uses is in the treatment of arthritis and rheumatism, as it improves the clearance of toxins from the system. The root tastes fairly bitter and acts as a central nervous system stimulant, probably through its action on the vagus nerve, though the tea of the root is more oily and aromatic than bitter. It has been used as a liver stimulant and as a tonic for the gall bladder.

As an oily, nutritive plant, I tend to use it for dry conditions, where the lack of oil in the system is causing cells and tissues to dry out – so it is particularly good for those who feel that their joints or muscles are drying out. The root is better suited for chronic conditions, and the seed for acute problems. The seed is also more suited to the skin and kidneys and has a much more diffusive flavour to it (if you can get past the problems involved with preparing it!)

For women's issues, the root has been used to regulate the menstrual cycle and is a gentle uterine stimulant. It has been used to treat uterine prolapse and also as a tonic to strengthen the womb before and after birth.

The fresh root is antibacterial and antifungal, and it can help the body regulate blood sugar levels – another good reason to include it in the diet and as a medicine.

**Folklore**    There are a few pieces of folklore associated with the plant, although very little folklore is known overall. The plant seems to have remained relatively unknown throughout history, although its Latin name – *Arctium* – comes from the Latin *Arctos*, meaning "bear". This is probably due to the hairy appearance of the well-known burrs. Two of the common names of the plant – "personata" and "prosopium" – come from the Greek and Latin names for "masked", because historically the large leaves were used as masks by Greek actors. The Native American Indians make extensive use of the plant as a vasotonic alterative. The young leaves were eaten as spring salads in Italy, Scandinavia and parts of France.

**Dose**    Dosage is generally 6 ml of tincture or 4 g of dried plant matter in an infusion. If you are using the seed tincture, I tend to suggest no more than 5 drops twice a day, as it can be rather strong and in large doses will precipitate a healing crisis.

**Contraindications**    Better used in smaller doses. Larger doses increase removal of toxins from the body and can cause a healing crisis. The plant is part of the Asteraceae family, which can cause skin reactions in some people. Not advised for use during pregnancy due to uterine stimulant effects.

# Burdock recipes

## Dandelion and burdock drink

**Ingredients**
- » fresh or dried dandelion root – at least 1 tbsp heaped
- » fresh or dried burdock root – as above
- » 1 organic lemon
- » fresh root ginger
- » cinnamon – ½ tsp (2.5 g)
- » raw cane sugar, maple syrup or local honey to taste
- » 1.2 l (40 fl oz) of water

**Instructions**    Remove the zest from the lemon, chop it finely, and pop it into a pan with the water and the cleaned and chopped roots and spices. Add the lemon juice and bring the whole lot to a gentle simmer for at least 20 minutes, or until it has reduced down by one third. Strain out the herbs and add the sweetener (sugar, syrup or honey) to taste. Drink half a cup twice a day as a general-purpose liver and lymph tonic. This is a really great spring drink to wake the body back up, as well as a good all-purpose liver tonic. You could also add a few handfuls of nettles and cleavers to add an extra lymphatic and all-round mineral kick! This recipe will keep for a week in the fridge, so I suggest making small batches regularly rather than one large batch. If you want to keep the mixture for longer, try freezing it in ice-cube trays and taking out a couple of cubes as needed.

## Burdock seed tincture

**Ingredients**
- » plenty of burdock seed heads
- » vodka

**Instructions**     Gather the seed heads in late summer, once they have gone brown – I'd advise not using a cloth bag for these, as the little claws on the seed heads will grab hold of the fabric and are very difficult to get free of the bag afterwards. They will also hook into skin with great abandon – another issue to be aware of during preparation. The seed heads will need to be put into a plastic bag and given a good bashing to get the seeds to drop free of the protective casings. Once you have encouraged them to let go of their fixings, you can use a mortar and pestle to give them a good bashing to break the surfaces down. Pile them into a Kilner jar and pour over plenty of vodka to cover the seeds, shaking the mixture up every other day. Store it in a cool, dark cupboard and let it steep for at least a month to allow the alcohol to get the best out of the seeds, then filter the remaining tincture through a coffee filter paper to remove any remaining hairs. The resulting tincture can be taken in drop doses of 5 drops twice a day for skin and kidney issues.

## Burdock root elixir

**Ingredients**
- » one decent chunk of burdock root – this is really flexible depending on the size of the piece you have managed to unearth
- » brandy
- » honey

**Instructions**    Scrub the root clean as much as you can, using a small paring knife to remove little side shoots and any damaged bits of root where the soil is too ingrained to remove it easily. Finely chop the root, or grate it if you can, as this will really break the root down thoroughly. Pile it into a jar and pour over enough alcohol to cover the root, then add a spoonful of honey if you want a sweet elixir. Leave the honey out if you would prefer a straight-up tincture. Put the lid on and let the whole lot steep for a month, then strain out the root before bottling the tincture or elixir. Take ½ tsp (2.5 ml) doses up to twice a day as a tonic.

# Calamus

## *Acorus calamus*

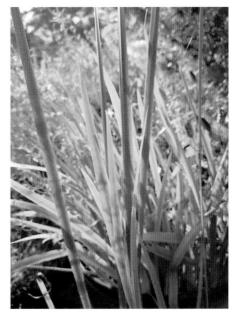

*Also known as:*   sweet flag, gladdon, myrtle grass, cinnamon sedge, sweet sedge

**Family**   Acoraceae.

**Habitat and description**   Calamus is a reed-like plant that thrives in marshy or watery soil, loving best of all the edges of ponds and slow-moving streams or rivers. I have also grown calamus very satisfactorily in a large pot with no piercings in the base, so it can be cultivated at home, though I suspect this method won't result in quite the same level of tasty constituents in it. Calamus grows up to 1 m (3¼ ft) tall and can colonise significant tracts of stream or pond bank, given half a chance, producing tall, sword-shaped leaves much like those of yellow or blue flag, though somewhat narrower. The rhizome is the part used in medicine, and it grows as a central, knobbly mass about as thick as a middle finger, with many smaller roots coming off it.

**Where to find it**    North America and Europe, where it can be found in parts of France, Germany, Scandinavia, and parts of the UK.

**Parts used**    The rhizome and roots.

**When to gather**    Late autumn or early spring, once the plant has reached a good size.

**Medicines to make**    Tinctures, elixirs and decoctions; honey and honegars.

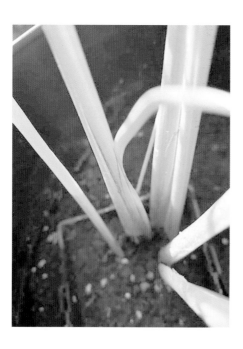

**Constituents**   Bitter volatile oils, including pinene and galangin; terpenes, including humulene; tannins, resins and mucilage.

**Planetary influence**   Unclassified, though, given its associations, I'm inclined to think possibly Jupiter.

**Associated deities and heroes**   None known at present, although it is more likely to be linked to Native American spirits, as it has not seen a long history of use in the UK.

**Festival**   None known at present.

**Constitution**   Warm and dry.

**Actions and indications**   Predominantly known and used as a digestive tonic, calamus root has a long history of use in North America; the plant was only brought to the UK in around 1560, by John Gerard. It has nevertheless developed a reputation for being an aromatic and carminative tonic, excellent for the relief of flatulent colic and dyspepsia, poor appetite and weight loss linked with anorexia. I have used it successfully to treat a damp, over-relaxed digestive tract leading to flatulence with abdominal griping and twisting pains, where it has warmed and toned the system remarkably quickly.

Calamus root also has some links with the lungs and the voice and makes an excellent cough remedy and antibacterial for infected chest conditions, especially where a lot of phlegm is being produced. I have used it with great success to help trauma survivors rediscover their voice – it is particularly useful for those who feel as though a hand is around their throat, removing their ability to speak and express their feelings. This can be a major stumbling block when trying to heal, and calamus root, used in small doses, often seems to have near-miraculous effects on this sort of issue. Calamus root also restores the voice where it has been over-strained by public speaking, singing or spending time in a smoky room, and it also facilitates speech when silence is the result of trauma. Calamus root is literally the hand helping us to see a way out of the murky depths of our own wounds. It is gently sedative to the central nervous system, so while it helps with speech, it also gently helps calm the whole system, so that experiences can be analysed more easily. It provides clarity and calm.

Calamus root has also been used to treat feverish conditions in those living in fen country, which is notorious for having a very damp climate with a lot of fog or mist. This is another example of the medicine plant to treat a problem growing near the cause of that problem – calamus grows very happily in the damp ground of fen country.

In parts of Asia, calamus root is given as a memory aid. In India, it is given ritually to newborns to improve intellect and encourage good speech development. In China, it is given after a stroke, to restore neural pathways and help concentration and focus.

**Folklore**    Historically, calamus leaves were used as a strewing herb in Norwich Cathedral, because of the scent of tangerines given off by the bruised herb. It grows very readily in Norfolk and Suffolk and was transported at great expense as far afield as London, for strewing in the churches there. The root and herb have been used in perfumery. The flowering spathe gives out quite a bit of heat, making the temperature around the plants noticeably warmer than further afield.

**Dose**    A small piece of root around the size of the little fingernail, and about 2 mm thick, chewed up to three times a day. Of the tincture, 1 tbsp (15 ml) in one week's worth of medicine is plenty. I generally suggest making a tincture in vodka, 2 ml of which to be taken up to three times a day for short periods of time.

**Contraindications**    Some members of the family contain reputedly cancer-encouraging oils, so do only use it for short

periods of time. This is another of the herbs that is a medicine, not a tonic, so do use it accordingly. Use with caution in
the case of buried trauma – taking the head off the volcano
can sometimes be more damaging than healing, so if you
are considering it for this purpose, ensure you have a good
support-network handy, including a therapist you trust.

# Calamus root recipes

## Calamus root honey

**Ingredients**
- » 1 jar of local honey
- » fresh calamus roots – as many as you want to unearth,
  without decimating the local population

**Instructions**   Thoroughly scrub and finely chop the calamus
roots into little pieces no larger than your little fingernail, or
grate the root on the largest grater setting. Put the chopped
pieces into a jar and then pour over a whole jar of local
honey, stirring carefully to submerge all the pieces. Pop the
lid on. These can be taken out and chewed as needed, or the
honey can be taken in 1 tsp (5 ml) doses to get the warming, stomachic properties into your system. Calamus root
is best taken cold, not heated, so I don't advise stirring it
into tea.

## Calamus root tincture

**Ingredients**
- » fresh calamus roots
- » vodka or brandy

**Instructions**    As with the above recipe, thoroughly scrub and chop the roots, then pile them into a wide-necked jar and pour over plenty of vodka, allowing an extra couple of centimetres on top. Let the whole lot macerate for at least a fortnight – I tend to suggest more like a month for roots and other tough plant parts. Strain out the roots after this time and compost them, and then bottle the tincture. Take 1 tsp (5 ml) up to three times a day for impaired digestion. Use short-term only – no more than a week, with two weeks between dosage periods.

## Storing fresh calamus root

To store fresh calamus root so that you can thaw it easily over the winter, scrub and finely chop the fresh roots, then spread them out on a tray and put it into the freezer. Every half an hour or so, take the tray out and give it a quick shake to stop the roots from sticking to it, then pop it back in again. Once they are fully frozen in separate small pieces, pour them into a freezer-suitable pot or bag, label them carefully, and put them back into the freezer. You can take out a few pieces as needed and thaw them out for chewing in order to freshen the breath and ease wind, bloating and indigestion.

# Chicory
## *Chicorium intybus*

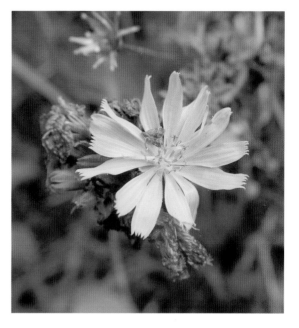

*Also known as:*   succory, wild succory, laidron, wegwarte

**Family**   Asteraceae.

**Habitat and description**   Chicory is a rather stately perennial that grows happily by the wayside, in meadows and on verges, reaching heights of over a metre (3¼ feet) in some places. In spring, the plant forms a brilliant green basal rosette of slightly hairy, green leaves that are shaped a little like those of a dandelion, with toothing and indentations running around the edges of long leaves. Later these leaves give rise to tall, tough, somewhat straggly stems with few leaves on, crowned with flowers much like those of the dandelion, but brilliant blue in colour, like the summer sky on a clear day. Swathes of this lovely plant grow by the roadsides in my native county of Lincolnshire, looking very much like the sky come down to earth, especially on more overcast days, when the blue colour is even clearer. The leaves that cling to the stems are more smooth-edged than the basal leaves and are scantily spaced up the stalk. The plant flowers generally from July to September, with the flowers closing by mid-afternoon when the sun is at its highest, a habit that has given rise to several different fairy-tales.

**Where to find it**    Most of the UK, where it prefers sandy, chalky or fairly light soils; Europe, where it was grown as a fodder crop for a while; parts of Scandinavia; parts of North America, where it has naturalised.

**Parts used**    Leaves, roots, seeds and flowers.

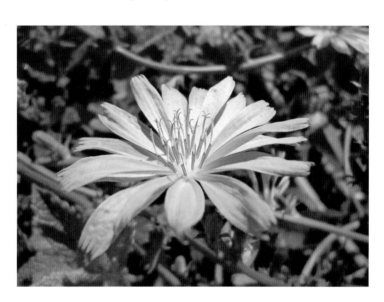

**When to gather**    Leaves, seeds and flowers in the summer and early autumn; root in winter.

**Medicines to make**    Decoctions and tinctures; syrups and honeys; poultices and plaisters; teas and flower waters.

**Constituents**    Inulin and sugars; alkaloids and flavonoids; sesquiterpene lactones and bitter glycosides responsible for the laxative and some of the digestive effects; triterpenes and coumarins.

**Planetary influence**    Jupiter.

**Associated deities and heroes**    Harvest deities. It is at its very best during harvest, where it can sometimes be found living in unsprayed corn and wheat fields.

**Festival**    Lammas.

**Constitution**    Cool and moist.

**Actions and indications**    The leaves, not as commonly used but considerably easier to gather than the root, have a fair few medicinal uses, including to relieve jaundice and to act as an all-round digestive tonic. They can also be pulverised as a poultice for a variety of skin issues including boils and abscesses, and many other inflamed skin conditions.

The root can be taken as a liver remedy, to detoxify and improve the health of the liver and spleen. It can also be used to relieve gallstones, preferably before they become large enough to become a real issue – take chicory if you have a history of developing gallstones, in order to prevent them becoming a problem again in the future. As an anti-inflammatory, it can be used to relieve inflammation in the digestive tract, as well as being hypoglycaemic – the presence of inulin in the root helps the body to better regulate blood sugar levels. This can also be of benefit in cases of fatty liver and liver inflammation, where it will gently reduce the inflammation and boost liver function back to normal levels. In this instance it is most effective when also combined with dietary changes.

Chicory is an excellent digestive tonic, helping the body to better make use of food products, to absorb minerals and molecules that are needed and to excrete the rest, making it a good food post-convalescence, and for those struggling with impaired digestion where this is affecting nerve endings and general levels of wellbeing. Well suited to phlegm in the digestive tract, chicory will help the body to remove excess phlegm so that the digestive system is better able to function. The antibacterial properties in the root make it of benefit in helping the body settle after food poisoning, where it acts as a tonic, kills off any remaining nasty bacteria, and helps the stomach settle back down to normal. Lastly, it can be very effective in the treatment of headaches, where digestive impairment is a strong feature. Keep track of how the stomach is functioning if you get regular cluster headaches that move from one side to the other – the digestive system features a plethora of nerve endings, and bloating and discomfort in the stomach can easily refer up to the head. Chicory can be used alongside angelica and blue flag for this purpose.

The root also has some effect on the bladder and kidneys, where it can increase and improve the removal of uric acid from the system, making it helpful by extension for the treatment of gout and rheumatism. Consider combining it with lymph remedies for these issues, to better encourage the removal of rubbish from around the joints. Use it also for water retention, as the diuretic properties help the body remove excess water without damaging the sodium and potassium balance that is vital for homeostasis.

The flowers have traditionally been extracted into a flower water and used to treat eye problems, including conjunctivitis. A tea of the flowers can be used for the same purpose.

**Folklore**    Chicory has been eaten as a vegetable for many hundreds of years, with the leaves being eaten by the Romans. Even today, chicory is cultivated as a root for grinding up as a coffee substitute, for which it is rather good.

There are two particular old folk tales about chicory that are very much linked with the eyes. According to one, chicory was originally a maiden who watched at the side of the road for her lover to return from war and was eventually turned into chicory to allow her to rest, as he never came back. Another features the beautiful, vain and unkind daughter of a witch, who spurned the sun in an unnecessarily rude fashion and was turned to chicory as a result and doomed to watch the sun for all eternity. Her witch mother intervened and managed to dull down the curse somewhat, allowing the flowers to close during the hottest part of the day. Interesting that both of these mention the affinity of the flowers with eyes, and the habit of the plant to grow by the side of the road.

**Dose**    Of the decoction, 2 tbsp (or approx. 30 ml) to be taken twice to three times a day. Tincture dosage up to 1 tsp (5 ml) twice a day.

**Contraindications**    None known at present.

# Chicory recipes

## *Chicory flower tea for eye inflammation*

### Ingredients / equipment
 » up to 10 chicory flower heads
 » hot water
 » coffee filter paper
 » one or two cotton-wool pads, or soft towelling pads for the eyes

**Instructions**   Shred the flowers into a cup and pour over a mug of hot water just off the boil. Let steep until cool, then strain out the flowers. Pour the resulting tea through a coffee filter paper to remove any bits that may irritate the eyes. Soak clean cotton wool pads in the tea, squeeze out some of the excess, and use them as eye compresses. You can also use this as an eye bath – pour a little of the tea into a clean eye-bath pot and use as needed to relieve inflammation and conjunctivitis. Remember to use different eye baths for each eye, and if you are suffering from conjunctivitis, avoid rubbing both eyes with the same hand, as this will often encourage the spread of the infection to the unaffected eye.

## Chicory root decoction

**Ingredients**
- » one medium-sized piece of chicory root – aim for something around the length of your palm
- » 570 ml (20 fl oz) of water

**Instructions**   Uproot the chicory after a bit of rain, to make it easier to get at the roots. Scrub the root thoroughly, then chop it into small pieces – the smaller the better. Pile the root into a non-aluminium pan and pour over the water, then bring to a gentle simmer for an hour. This will make a decoction that should last for three days if stored in the fridge. If you want a more stable decoction, keep simmering it for several hours, topping the water up as needed. Once the liquid has reduced by about half, at the end of the hour's simmering, strain out the roots and bottle the decoction, storing it in the fridge. Take up to 2 tbsp (30 ml) three times a day as an all-round liver and digestive system tonic, to restore the stomach after food poisoning, and to settle the stomach in the case of digestive-related headaches.

## Chicory root coffee

**Ingredients**
- » as much chicory root as you can get your hands on – growing it yourself is a great idea, if possible
- » patience!

**Instructions**    Gather the root in the autumn – you may want to mark where the plants were while they are above ground, just in case they have gone completely dormant by the time you want to make the coffee. Scrub the chicory root thoroughly and then cut into small pieces approximately 5 mm squared and around 3 mm thick. These small pieces then need to be dried out – either put them in a dehydrator until they are fully dried, or on a tray in a sunny place if you have a room that is a real sun trap and gets suitably warm. Once the roots have dried down completely, you can roast them in the oven. I tend to go for a moderate temperature of around 150°C, as my oven runs a little on the hot side, but experiment until you find a temperature that works for you. Let the root pieces roast slowly and steadily until they are a rich brown colour, then allow them to cool. These can be ground up using a mortar and pestle and then used to make coffee in much the usual way – just allow 1 dessertspoonful (around 8 g) of powder to a mug of hot water. Cafetieres work well here – just make the chicory root coffee in the same way as you would regular coffee.

# Comfrey
## *Symphytum officinale*

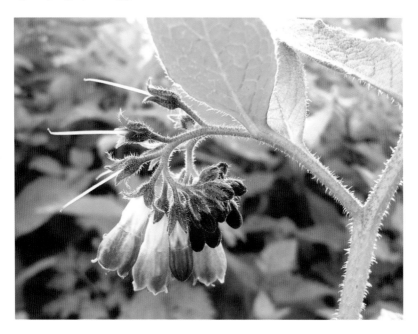

*Also known as:* knitbone, boneset (not to be confused with American boneset – *Eupatorium perfoliatum*), knitback, consound, blackwort, bruisewort, slippery root, yalluc (Saxon), gum plant, consolida, ass ear

**Family** Boraginaceae.

**Habitat and description** Comfrey rather likes to grow in damp, marshy soil, though it will do perfectly well in ordinary garden soil and can easily be grown as a garden plant. It can often be found on allotments, where it is grown as plant food and has a reputation for being a garden escapee and a bit of a thug. The flowers are small and bell-shaped, usually white or

56

pink in colour, uncurling from tight spirals to form in graceful arches at the top of a stem that tends to be thick and covered with quite prickly hairs. The leaves begin small but soon reach substantial proportions and are roughly spear-shaped and covered with the same prickly hairs as the stem. The plant grows up to a metre (3¼ feet) in height and will happily sprawl over half the garden if given a chance – if it starts to get too big, gather the leaves and make it into plant food, as it will happily nurture the rest of your garden when combined with nettle leaves: stinky, but good! The root is long, thick and juicy and difficult to get rid of, once you have it in the garden – be aware that you will need to dig deep to remove it in its entirety. If you don't want it to turn into a garden thug, try growing it in large pots instead.

**Where to find it**  Comfrey grows easily in most temperate countries of the world, including North America, Europe, western Asia and Australia.

**Parts used**  Comfrey root, rhizome and leaf are all used in herbal medicine.

**When to gather**  Leaves in summer; root and rhizome from October until November.

**Medicines to make**  Infused oils, teas, small quantities of young leaves steamed as a vegetable; poultice of the leaves. Concern about the pyrrolizidine alkaloid content makes me hesitant to recommend it as a tincture – some sources say that the pyrrolizidine alkaloid  content does not extract as well in water, so tea may be a safer way to use it. Regarding the safety of tea versus tincture, it is up to the reader to do further research to determine the most appropriate method of delivery.

**Constituents**  Comfrey contains around 4.7% allantoin (responsible for the healing effects), pyrrolizidine alkaloids (in the fresh young leaves and roots), mucilage, phenolic acids, steroidal saponins (root) and triterpenoids. Allantoin is a cell-proliferant, which accounts for comfrey's action in the healing of damaged tissue. The rosmarinic acid and other phenolic acids are responsible for its anti-inflammatory action. Pyrrolizidine alkaloids are highly toxic to the liver as isolated substances.

**Planetary influence**   Saturn.

**Associated deities and heroes**   The Goddess in her aspect of the Crone – that is, Hecate, Cerridwen; Death Goddesses, such as Inanna.

**Festival**   Samhain.

**Constitution**   Cold and moist.

**Actions and indications**   Comfrey has a well-deserved reputation as a wound healer, due to the presence of allantoin in the herb, speeding the healing of sprains, strains and broken bones, and also being a useful local treatment for minor cuts and grazes. Care must be taken when using this herb with deeper cuts or any wound that may not be fully clean, because it speeds the healing to the point where it can cause abscesses

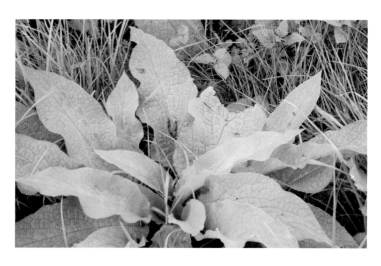

in deeper wounds, as the top heals before the bottom of the wound does. This is particularly important if the wound still has dirt trapped in it. The herb can be used topically for sprains, fractures, torn ligaments, crush injuries and related strains and sprains, either as an infused oil or as a poultice, but again the presence of allantoin can cause broken bones to heal too rapidly, causing bony nodules to build over the break site. It is better used once the bone has knit cleanly. The herb can also be used as a water wash to slow the progression of psoriasis.

The plant can be used to treat hot, dry conditions of the gut, such as dyspepsia (acid indigestion), peptic ulcers and irritable bowel syndrome. It combines very well with meadowsweet as a tea for peptic ulceration, where it has the action of balancing acid levels as well as healing ulceration. It is antispasmodic, and the mucilage in it forms a protective coating over the lining of the stomach, cooling and soothing and encouraging healing. The plant has astringent qualities, so it can be used to treat haemorrhage, where again the allantoin content can heal damaged mucous membrane surfaces. The demulcent properties can also be used to soothe lung troubles and coughs, though again use with caution because of the pyrrolizidine alkaloids content; hot or cold infusion is your best bet, and a cold infusion will pull out far more of the mucilage if it is the soothing action you are after.

**Folklore**   The alternative common names "knitbone" and "consolida" indicate that this plant has a long history of use on injuries. The name comfrey derives from the words con firma, meaning to unite. The herb was written about by the Greek physician Dioscorides in the first century ce. The fresh leaves can be used as a vegetable as they contain vitamin B12, and are the only vegetable sources of this vitamin. The plant itself can be used as a natural fertilizer if left in water for several months. It combines particularly well with nettle for this purpose, though the combination is rather smelly!

**Dose**    One teaspoon of fresh or dried herb to a cup of hot water, steeped for 5 minutes and sipped, twice a day. Cold infusion: fresh herb finely chopped and steeped overnight in cold water. Again, one cup twice a day for short periods of time. Short-term use only is advised due to the pyrrolizidine alkaloid content, as pyrrolizidine alkaloids are highly toxic to the liver as isolated substances.

**Contraindications**    Comfrey ointment should never be used over the top of deep or dirty wounds, as it may cause the formation of abscesses. The herb should not be taken during pregnancy or while breastfeeding. Avoid using comfrey internally for any reason if you have a history of liver ill health.

# Comfrey recipes

## Comfrey salve for bruises, bumps, strains and sprains

### Ingredients
- » 8 large comfrey leaves, in two batches of 4 leaves each
- » organic seed oil, such as rapeseed, sweet almond or sunflower
- » beeswax pellets
- » rosemary and mint essential oils

**Instructions**    Make sure the surface of the leaves is completely dry, then finely chop them in a food processor, or by hand using kitchen scissors or a mezzaluna. Pile them into the top of a double boiler and pour over enough oil to just cover the leaves, then put them onto a moderate heat, making sure there is water in the bottom of the pan. Let them steep for at least half an hour, then strain out the herbs through kitchen roll, before repeating the process with the second lot of fresh leaves. Once the second lot have infused, strain out the oil through some kitchen roll and add 12 g of beeswax to 100 ml (3½ fl oz) of oil. Make sure the top of the double boiler has been given a good wipe to remove shreds of leaf, then put the oil and beeswax back in, letting the whole lot heat through gently until the wax has melted. Stir it, then add 5 drops each of rosemary and mint essential oils per 100 ml (3½ fl oz) of salve mixture. Stir again quickly, then pour it into clean jars, putting the lid on once the mixture has cooled slightly.

This balm can be used for bruises, bumps, strains and sprains, but do not use it on open wounds, cuts or scrapes.

## Comfrey, meadowsweet and marshmallow leaf tea for peptic ulcers and indigestion

**Ingredients**
- » 2 tbsp of dried comfrey leaf
- » 2 tbsp of dried meadowsweet leaves
- » 2 tbsp of dried marshmallow leaves

**Instructions**   Meadowsweet and marshmallow leaves can be dried by hanging them up in bunches or piling them into trays until they have dried down, but comfrey is a bit more tricky. Because the leaves rot so quickly, you will need either a dehydrator or a very low oven to get them to dry as quickly as you can – I don't advise trying to dry them naturally, as you will be woken up in the small hours of the morning by the most unbelievable stench. Make sure the leaves are completely dehydrated before you blend this tea, or they will rot and ferment in the jar – remember the aforementioned stench as a suitable deterrent!

Once the leaves are all completely dry, finely chop them using kitchen scissors and mix them together thoroughly in a decent-sized bowl, then pile them into a clean, dry jar, labelling it with the date, the ingredients and the purpose of the blend. Use 1 tsp to a cup of just-off-the-boil water, steeping the mixture for 5 minutes before drinking. Take twice a day to encourage the lining of the stomach to heal swiftly and acid levels to begin to balance out. Use with caution in the case of a previous history of liver ailments.

## Comfrey and nettle plant food

**Ingredients**
- » plenty of nettles and comfrey leaves and stems
- » enough water to cover the plant matter
- » a large bucket with a tight-fitting lid
- » a peg (for your nose, while it is brewing!)

**Instructions**    Roughly chop or shred the leaves if you can – you can put them into a pile and use a fairly sharp garden spade to chop them up if you want, and this often saves quite a bit of time. Pile the ingredients into the bucket and pour over enough water to cover the herbs, then put the lid on. Put the bucket in an out-of-the-way place until it has had time to brew up – this usually takes around three weeks to a month to really get the best out of it. If you can get a brewing bucket with a tap in the bottom for this, so much the better, as it will make decanting off some of the smelly garden food a lot easier. To use the feed, just add half a pint of the plant food to a 20-litre (4.5-gallon) can of water and use it to water the plants. This food works beautifully for vegetables like tomatoes as well – just feed the plants once or twice a week once the first truss of fruits has set.

# Cramp bark
*Viburnum opulus*

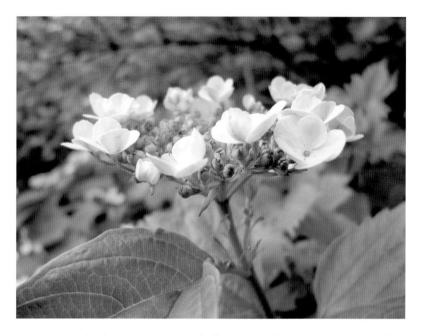

*Also known as:* snowball tree, Guelder rose, rose elder, silver
bells, king's crown, Whitsun rose, high cranberry, May rose

**Family**   Caprifoliaceae.

**Habitat and description**   This handsome little shrub is commonly used here in the UK as a hedging plant and is a welcome
sight indeed in spring, when it is adorned with clusters of
creamy flowers. The flowers themselves form an unusual pattern, called a corymb, with a ring of larger outer flowers, which
are sterile, and a cluster of much smaller, fertile flowers in
the centre – these are much visited by insects. In autumn the
berries form, which, when ripe, are a translucent red colour,
much beloved of birds and small beasties. The shrub itself

grows up to 2.5 m (8 ft) tall if given enough room without regular pruning, and it features woody stems that play host to a plethora of beautiful lobed leaves, which usually have three main lobes and some lesser toothing around the edges. These turn red and purple tones in autumn, making a very fetching display indeed in the hedgerows, especially when the slightly translucent, brilliant scarlet berries play counterpart to them.

**Where to find it**    A common hedging plant, cramp bark can be found around the UK, as well as in North America, where it is indigenous. Also found across parts of Europe and as far away as Russia.

**Parts used**    Predominantly the bark, but also the berries, have been used as an ingredient in cooking, hence the name "high cranberry".

**When to gather**    The bark can be gathered year-round. The berries can be gathered in the autumn.

**Medicines to make**    Syrups, tinctures and elixirs; dried bark for decoctions.

**Constituents**    Bitter glycosides including viburnine. Tannins and resins. Coumarins and hydroquinones, and valerianic acid, which is responsible for the relaxant properties found in the plant.

**Planetary influence**    None allocated – cramp bark only has

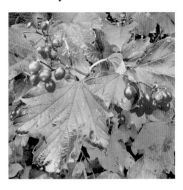 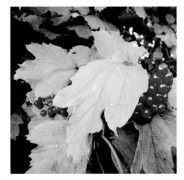

a documented history of use dating back 400 years, which is comparatively short compared to many other herbs and might be why it has not yet been associated with any planets.

**Associated deities and heroes**　No known deities or heroes at the present time.

**Festival**　Lammas.

**Constitution**　Cool and dry.

**Actions and indications**　Cramp bark is not considered to be as strong as its relative, black haw (V. prunifolium), but the latter is not really available in the UK for growing in the medicine garden, nor have I found it in the hedgerows, as it generally doesn't thrive outside the east coast of North America. Black haw has a particular affinity with the uterus and the menstrual cycle, although I generally use cramp bark as a general-purpose antispasmodic.

Cramp bark has a wide range of uses in herbal medicine. One of the main areas in which it is of particular value is in the treatment of spasmodic cramps throughout the body, including smooth muscle cramps of the digestive system, as well as tension headaches, where its gentle nervine balancing properties also come into play. As an extension of this, it can also be used to relieve anxiety and hysteria, particularly where this is linked to cramping and spasm of the digestive organs.

While not as strong as black haw, it can also be used to relieve menstrual cramping and heavy bleeding and has been used to stop threatened miscarriage, as well as acting as a partus preparator before labour.

The herb is also a handy addition to remedies and recipes linked with the heart and vascular system and can be used with other herbs to relieve high blood pressure, especially where this is due to tension within the blood vessels themselves, and to relieve other vascular disorders. Use it to relieve angina and palpitations, as well as intermittent claudication.

The kidneys and bladder can also benefit from cramp bark, as it will relieve spasm and allow smoother functioning of the kidneys, allowing better filtration and excretion.

Cramp bark can also be combined with other ingredients in the treatment of rheumatism and arthritis, as well as polymyalgia – any issues where there is spasming and cramping of the muscles.

The valerianic acid in cramp bark also contributes to a gentle sedative action. The flavour of the tincture is startlingly fragrant, almost like perfume.

**Folklore**    The berries are used as a substitute for cranberries in Canada. The name "Guelder" comes from the original region of Holland where the tree was first properly cultivated for hedging and as a garden plant. In areas of Siberia and Scandinavia the berries are used for a variety of purposes, including as part of a spirit, and mixed into pastes with flour and honey. Viburnum is one of the national symbols of the Ukraine, where it is also linked with the old Slavic pagan religions of the region. The symbol can often be found on clothing and jewellery from the area.

**Dose**    1 tsp (5 ml) of the tincture up to three times a day.

**Contraindications**    Consuming too many of the berries can cause vomiting.

# Cramp bark recipes

## Cramp bark elixir for spasms and nervous headaches

**Ingredients**
» several decent-sized twigs from a cramp bark shrub – go for 25 cm (10 in.) lengths if possible, and get at least three of them

» 2 tbsp of German chamomile flowers
» 6 stems of lemon balm, or 3 tbsp of the dried herb
» brandy
» honey or maple syrup

**Instructions**    First, use a paring knife to strip the bark off the twigs, peeling away from yourself and getting as much of the inner bark as you can. Once you have stripped off the bark, use a pair of kitchen scissors to cut it into small pieces and pack them into a Kilner jar, then add the other herbs, chopped if fresh. Pour over plenty of brandy to cover the herbs, with a centimetre on top, and add as much honey or maple syrup as you prefer. Let the whole thing steep for four weeks, shaking it up every other day. At the end of this time, strain out the herbs and bottle the resulting elixir. Take 1 tsp (5 ml) every couple of hours, up to four doses in a day. Use it to relieve stress and tension in all its forms, particularly when this causes headaches or upset stomach.

## Cramp bark tonic for circulation

**Ingredients**
» several 25 cm (10 in.) pieces of cramp bark shrub stem
» ½ pint of hawthorn berries – fresh, if possible
» 6 stems of fresh yarrow flowering tops
» 3 tbsp of dried limeflowers
» 1 tbsp of dried elderflowers
» brandy or vodka as preferred

**Instructions**    As with the previous recipe, strip the bark and finely chop it, then pile it into a Kilner jar, along with the rest of the herbs, making sure that the yarrow is finely chopped. Don't bruise the hawthorn berries though, or they will make your tonic solidify! Pour in the alcohol, allowing an extra couple of centimetres on top of the herbs. Let the whole lot steep for a month, then strain out the herbs. Take 1 tsp (5 ml) twice a day to relieve early symptoms of high blood pressure, and as a tonic for Raynaud's disease. If the high blood pressure is due to stress, consider adding chamomile, lemon balm and skullcap to the tonic blend.

# Elecampane
## *Inula helenium*

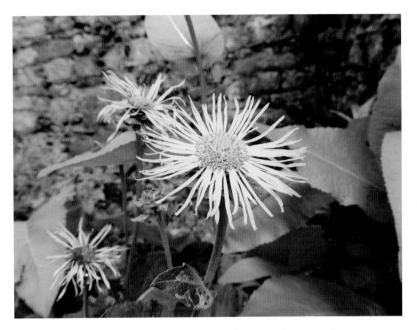

*Also known as:* marchalan, elfwort, scabwort, yellow starwort, spearwort, wallwort, elfdock, horseheal, velvet dock, wild sunflower, alycompaine, enula, alantwurzel, aunee

**Family** Asteraceae.

**Habitat and description** Our tall, sunny friend elecampane grows up to 2½ m tall (over 8 ft) in good conditions, with large oval leaves growing in alternate pairs on a robust, sturdy stem. The leaves themselves are rough-textured on the upper surface and fluffy underneath, with some hairs growing on the stem as well: they feature a beautiful, intricate pattern of veins that is well worth a closer look. The root grows fairly deep and is moist and juicy when cut. As with most roots, it should be gathered in the autumn, in the second year of growth. The flowers are large and look rather like those of a daisy, but are bright yellow – they grow during the hottest part of the year and are a glorious sight, though the stems can get rather bashed about by late summer storms.

Elecampane grows happily on waste ground and by the wayside, preferring to grow near human dwellings – perhaps another reason why the Anglo-Saxons used it to treat illnesses caused by 'elf arrows' – sudden, sharp pains or ailments thought to be caused by bolts shot by unseen elves. Elecampane prefers moist, fertile soil but will grow on less well favoured ground as well, provided that it has plenty of sun. The plant is best used fresh, as much of the medicinal content comes from the volatile oils, which are only present in the fresh root – so fresh root should be used, or a tincture made from the fresh root.

**Where to find it**   Europe, Asia and North America, where it has been a traditional member of medicine gardens for hun-

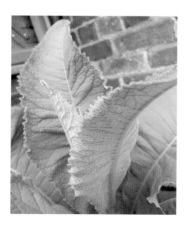
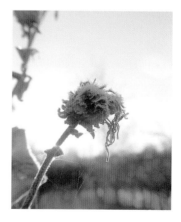

dreds of years, towering happily over pretty much every other denizen, as well as being significantly taller than most, if not all, human visitors.

**Parts used**    Root, leaves.

**When to gather**    Late autumn and early winter.

**Medicines to make**    Tinctures, syrups and vinegars; grated root; infused oil of the leaves and root.

**Constituents**    Sesquiterpene lactones, triterpenes, sterols, mucilage, up to 44% inulin, resins, up to 4% volatile oils, and bitters including helenin – which is responsible in part for the plant's strongly antibacterial properties.

**Planetary influence**    Mercury.

**Associated deities and heroes**    Helen of Troy. I suspect this beauty can, by extension, also be associated with various faery deities, such as Titania and Mab. It has long had an association with elves.

**Festival**    Summer solstice / midsummer.

**Constitution**    Hot and dry.

**Actions and indications**    Elecampane is used predominantly for the lungs, especially to clear up toxic, wet conditions. It is a stimulating expectorant and is very heating, making it unsuitable for those who tend towards excessive heat – for example, those who overheat very easily and who don't tolerate hot temperatures well, have a more red complexion, and tend to get head rushes when they stand up. Small doses, however, are excellent for improving the health of lung tissue, resolving chronic, long-lasting coughs and lung complaints in which a lot of phlegm is produced, and for chest infections with a strong emotional component. Elecampane is a fantastic herb to use for chronic, longlasting infections that have led to the production of greenish-coloured mucus.

By extension, elecampane can be used to soothe and resolve fevers, in particular those caused by deep-seated infections, although again use with caution due to its heating effects.

Being a warming, aromatic, mild stimulant, the root can also be used to encourage the appetite, as well as being useful in toning up a lax, over-relaxed digestive tract, especially where a lot of mucus is present. It can be used in small quantities to relieve stomach ache as a result of post-nasal drip following a bad head cold. It is very good for resolving lymphatic stagnation surrounding the digestive system, where this has led to overproduction of mucus and insufficient absorption of nutrients from food, as well as for wind and intestinal spasms caused by hyper-relaxed membranes.

Topically, elecampane is one of the most antiseptic and antibacterial herbs that can be grown in the garden. It can be applied to wounds that refuse to scab over, and the oil can be used to soothe rheumatic pain worsened by cold.

Elecampane has also been used as a supportive agent when managing diabetes. Inulin, which, in addition to having a positive effect on gut bacteria health, has been shown to help the body to moderate insulin resistance and blood sugar balance, is certainly present in elecampane root. For the management of diabetes, elecampane combines well with dandelion root and cinnamon bark.

Elecampane root is well suited for those who have had a sudden emotional trauma – especially one caused by unexpected, massive life changes – and it can also be used to boost immune function. It is often sudden trauma after long periods of stress that triggers chronic fatigue syndrome (CFS) and is another indicator for it. Poor immune function is also characteristic of many CFS sufferers, so the use of elecampane seems indicated in these situations. Sufferers also may experience extreme temperature fluctuations, feeling either the cold or the heat intensely, and often have done so since well before their diagnosis of CFS. Also, improving the absorption of nutrients by the digestive tract is always a useful way to begin treating such a deep-seated illness.

**Folklore**   The second part of the Latin name for this plant, "*helenium*", is said to have been given to the plant after it grew where Helen of Troy's tears fell after she was abducted by Paris (depending, of course, on which version of the legend you've been told!). According to other tales, it was called "*helenium*" after the island Helena, where the best plants were said to have grown.

Elecampane was very well known by the Anglo-Saxons, who used it extensively both in medicine and to ward off the infamous afflictions caused by being elf-shot. Later it was also used by the Welsh physicians, who knew it as marchalan.

Use of elecampane dates back to the Greek physicians Galen and Hippocrates, and the saying "*Enula campana reddit praecordia sana*", or "Elecampane will sustain the spirits", comes from ancient Rome.

**Dose**   No more than 6 ml three times a day, though I would recommend less than this to start off with: as it is ruled by Mercury, you can never tell exactly how it will affect an individual.

**Contraindications**   Do not use during pregnancy or while breastfeeding.

# Elecampane recipes

## Elecampane for chest infections

### Ingredients
- » fresh elecampane root, as much as you have to work with
- » vodka or apple cider vinegar
- » honey

**Instructions**    There are three basic ways to preserve elecampane (that I prefer to use, anyway!). One is simply to clean and finely chop or grate the root, then freeze it on a tray in small pinches (no more than the size of a lentil). Shake the tray every now and then so that the root doesn't get stuck to it. These tiny frozen pinches of root can then be put into a ziploc bag and stored in the freezer. Just defrost them as you need them and chew them raw, if possible, to help your body to clear chest infections. Be aware that the root has quite some heat and pungency to it!

Another method is to steep the finely chopped root in either vinegar or vodka with some honey added, to make an elixir for chest infections. Leave the root in – if you need extra pep to your remedy, you can take a dose of the elixir and then fish out a little bit of the root and chew it for good measure.

The third method is to make elecampane honey.


## Elecampane honey

**Ingredients**
  » 1 large piece of fresh elecampane root
  » one or two jars of local honey – runny, if possible

**Instructions**    Finely chop or grate the fresh root and pile it into jars, then pour over the honey. Be aware that you will need to keep stirring up the honey every few days to ensure the elecampane both extracts into it and is preserved by it. Leave to infuse for at least a month before using. You can either chew small pieces of the root as they are, or add teaspoonfuls of the honey to medicinal teas. Sage tea, sweetened with elecampane, can be used for sore throats linked with chest infections.

## Elecampane plaister for sore joints

**Ingredients**
  » elecampane leaves and/or root
  » organic seed oil
  » beeswax
  » black pepper essential oil

**Instructions**  As with so many infused oil recipes, this requires the use of a double boiler. If you are using the root, scrub it clean and then let the surface completely dry before you progress any further with this recipe. Once the root is surface dry, it can be grated up and piled into the double boiler. Leaves can be chopped as they are and piled in. Pour over the oil, and let the whole lot infuse for at least an hour, preferably longer. Repeat the process with fresh ingredients after this time for a really strong oil. Strain out the herbs and add 16 g of beeswax per 100 ml (3½ fl oz) of oil, returning it to the heat until the wax has melted. Add 5 drops of black pepper essential oil per 100 ml (3½ fl oz) of the mixture, stir to mix it up thoroughly, and then pour the resulting salve over squares of cloth on dinner plates – old tea towels work well for this, cut into quarters. Once the plaisters have set, peel them off the plates and put them onto large squares of greaseproof paper. Scrape the remainder of the ointment off the plates and smear it onto the cloths as well, then fold the paper over the top of the plaister and roll it up. The rolled plaisters can be secured with rubber bands or twine and stored in a glass jar until needed. To use a plaister, unroll it and apply it to the sore joint in question, bandaging it in place. Wear scruffy clothes, just in case the ointment melts and drips. Try to leave the plaister in place for at least half an hour if possible.

To make a salve version of this, follow the recipe for the plaister but add 12 g of beeswax per 100 ml (3½ fl oz) of mixture, instead of 16 g. After adding the black pepper essential oil, stir the mixture well and pour the salve into clean glass jars. Label them carefully, and massage the salve into sore joints.

# Hawthorn / Midland hawthorn
## *Crataegus monogyna / Crataegus laevigata*

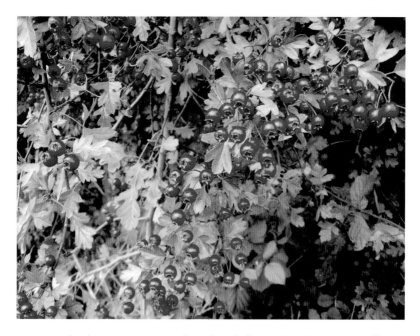

*Also known as:* may, bread and cheese, hagthorn, moon flower, whitethorn, quickthorn, may tree, mayblossom, ladies' meat, gaxels, halves, huath, may bush, mayflower, tree of chastity and quickset, chucky cheese, cuckoo's beads, pixie pears

**Family** Rosaceae. The name *Crataegus oxyacantha* is sometimes still used for hawthorn, although it has been rejected by the International Botanical Congress as being ambiguous.

**Habitat and description** Hawthorn is a familiar sight growing alongside paths and near rivers, as well as being widely used as a hedging plant in the countryside. It can often grow to 9 m (30 ft) tall. From the end of April onwards it has clusters of beautiful five-petalled white flowers with a musky odour. Some varieties sport pink flowers, others have deep mauve, double- or triple-petalled flowers. The tree can often be found growing near human habitation, and it provides food and shelter for many birds, small mammals and insects, making it an essential part of hedgerows.

Hawthorn leaves are deeply divided into toothed lobes, which are bright green when just out of bud but become shiny green on top and grey-green below once mature. The young buds can be eaten as a snack or used as an ingredient in salads and pesto. The fruit, also known as haws, are initially green in colour but gradually turn a rich, intense red; they are best gathered after a frost, as this makes the skins much softer. The berries have either one or two seeds depending on the species (*C. monogyna* has one seed, *C. laevigata* has two).

The tree can live to over 400 years old, and hawthorn remains found in megalithic tombs show that the tree was

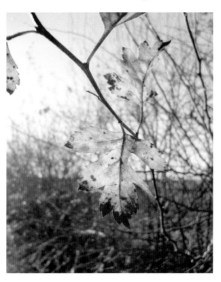

widespread around Britain before 6000 BCE. The scent of hawthorn is either loved or hated by most; some varieties have more of a vanilla scent, others more of a musky or even fishy scent.

**Where to find it**   Hawthorn can be found growing all over Europe, parts of Africa and Asia, and many other temperate regions of the world, where it is sometimes considered a weed.

**Parts used**   Leaves and flowering tops, berries.

**When to gather**   May for the flowering tops; September, October and November for the berries.

**Medicines to make**   Hawthorn flower elixir or tincture; hawthorn berry elixir, tincture or syrup; hawthorn fruit leather.

**Constituents**   Hawthorn contains flavonoids, including rutin, procyanidins and catechins; phenolic acids, including caffeic acid; amines; and triterpenes based on ursolic acid and oleanolic acid. The presence of rutin would seem to account at least in part for the plant's beneficial effect on the cardiovascular system. The leaves of *C. monogyna* have higher levels of flavonoids than do those of *C. laevigata*, although both varieties contain the oligomeric procyanidins responsible for the cardio-protective properties of the plant. Rutin, bioflavonoids and trimethylamine are found only in the flowers, whereas the berries have tannins, ascorbic acid, saponins and procyanidins. I tend to suggest that tincturing the flowers and berries separately is a good plan – make a 50/50 mix of the two individual tinctures afterwards for a whole-plant tincture.

**Planetary influence**   Mars.

**Associated deities and heroes**   Blodeuwedd, Cardea, Creiddylad, Fairies, Flora, Hymen, Olwen and Thor, as well as Govannon, Vulcan, Hephaestus, Mars and Hera.

**Festival**   Beltane.

**Constitution**    Cool and dry in the first degree – most herbalists tend to agree that the plant is slightly sour and cooling but is only gently refrigerant rather than being excessively cold.

**Actions and indications**    Hawthorn is primarily known as a heart and cardiovascular tonic, and is mainly used for this purpose today. It can also be used to scavenge and remove excess cholesterol from the blood vessels, making it a superb tonic food for anyone with a family history of heart problems or high cholesterol. Hawthorn berries can also be used as part of a healthy diet to promote long-term heart health.

The flowers, leaves and berries all have vasodilatory properties, which can be used to improve blood supply around the body. It is an excellent herb to use to treat high blood pressure when this is related to hardening of the arteries (arteriosclerosis), as well as being a useful tonic for poor memory and confusion caused by poor blood supply to the brain.

It has been used to treat angina, cardiac failure and conditions such as Raynaud's phenomenon, tachycardia and thrombosis, as well as venous problems such as intermittent claudication.

It can be used to prolong exercise duration and has been taken by sportsmen to sustain the heart during maximum physical effort – indeed, I advise it as a staple part of the diet for anyone doing sustained, intensive activity, whether it is weightlifting or endurance sports. It is a superb antioxidant, full of free-radical scavengers as well as the heart-healthy properties already mentioned.

Some herbalists even use it to reduce and even reverse age-related degeneration of the heart – we have so much of it growing in our hedgerows that I can't help but agree with this idea.

Hawthorn can be used to promote digestive function and to dissolve deposits and help weight loss. This is possibly due to its positive action on the heart and circulatory system, allowing optimum heart function and improved circulation, though it also has a powerful effect in terms of removing cholesterol from the arteries, as already mentioned – not too big a step, then, to believe that it could also affect long-stored patches and pockets of body fat.

**Folklore**     There is a wide body of folklore surrounding the hawthorn tree, dating back thousands of years. As it has traditionally always flowered around Beltane, throughout the month of May, it is associated with lust, fertility and sexuality and has always been connected to the Goddess in her guise as Maiden. This is particularly interesting given that this plant is often thought to be masculine in energy.

As previously mentioned, hawthorn is a faery tree and is one of the triad associated with the Fair Folk – oak, ash and (haw)thorn. To cut a branch from the hawthorn without asking the permission of the Fair Folk was said to bring great danger and ill fortune. The hawthorn is associated with witches, who are said to be able to turn themselves into hawthorn trees at will – this bears some resemblance to the similar legend attached to the elder (*Sambucus nigra*) and is probably not too surprising, given that elder and hawthorn growing together was considered to be nearly as powerful as the Faery Triad.

There is a longstanding belief that to bring hawthorn into the house is extremely unlucky unless this is done on Beltane, when cutting and bringing a branch of flowering hawthorn indoors is considered to bring the Goddess's blessing on the inhabitants of the house. Hawthorn was traditionally used to adorn the maypole as part of the Beltane festivities.

One of the earliest Goddesses associated with hawthorn was Olwen, also known as "She of the White Track" – as wherever she stepped, hawthorn sprang up in her tracks. This is certainly represented well by the hawthorn hedges that resemble white paths through fields when the tree is flowering.

Hawthorn wood is fine-grained and hard and is ideal for making small items such as knife handles. The wood burns readily and produces great heat, hot enough to melt iron when used in charcoal form.

Finally, there is, of course, the old legend that Joseph of Arimathea planted his hawthorn staff in the soil on Glastonbury Tor, where it rooted and produced flowers at rather odd times of the year – something that is, in fact, not so unusual, as hawthorn has been known to flower twice a year. Sadly, the original Glastonbury thorn was cut down by Cromwell's army, as the legend surrounding it was considered idolatry.

**Dose**    I tend to say that for an elixir, 2 tsp (10 ml) twice a day of the combined flower and berry elixir should be sufficient. For a tincture, I recommend 1 tsp (5 ml) a day.

**Contraindications**    Some herbalists reckon hawthorn cannot be used for low blood pressure, while others think it can be used perfectly safely for this. I would suggest that, if you do

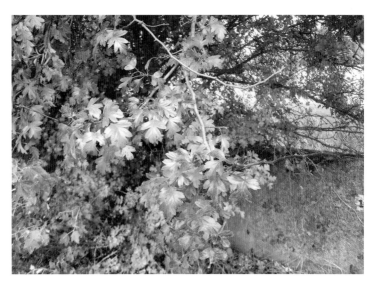

suffer from this, you use it carefully, check with your doctor and monitor your blood pressure.

# Hawthorn recipes

## Hawthorn berry syrup

**Ingredients**
- » 900 g (2 lb) of hawthorn berries or more
- » 1 whole lemon
- » 1.2 l (40 fl oz) of water
- » 1 kg (2 lb 3½ oz) of sugar – preferably organic or Fairtrade

**Instructions**  This syrup, although not exactly promising in scent while you make it, actually has a delicious flavour once cool, tasting rather like strawberry. It is made in much the same way as many fruit-based syrups. Start by lightly crushing the hawthorn berries, either by putting them into a clean polythene bag and bashing them with a rolling pin to break the surface of the berry skins, or by bashing them roughly in batches, using a mortar and pestle. I would recommend that you do not use a blender to crush them, as they contain stones that can get jammed under the blade. Another option is to freeze the berries overnight, as freezing does a nice job of breaking the skins down. Whichever method you choose, next put the slightly mangled or frozen berries into a pan, add the water and the juice and zest of the lemon, and bring to a boil. Simmer for 30 minutes, leave to cool, filter out the berries and add the sugar.

Bring the mixture back to the boil and simmer again until reduced down by about one third, then bottle the hot syrup, not forgetting to label the bottles. This syrup will keep for a long while in the fridge (up to six months, I find), and quite a long while outside it – three to six months, depending on where it has been stored.

## Hawthorn and apple ketchup

**Ingredients**
- » hawthorn berries, as many as you can bear to gather – around 400 g (14 oz) works well with the recipe quantities given
- » 2–3 apples – cooking apples are best
- » 1 large onion – red or white, depending on preference
- » as much garlic as you enjoy adding to recipes; I find that 2–5 cloves works well
- » 350 ml (12 fl oz) of red wine vinegar
- » salt to taste
- » oil for cooking – you can use oak-smoked rapeseed, garlic-infused, or whichever you prefer
- » Mediterranean herbs – oregano, rosemary and thyme work well
- » brown sugar to taste

**Instructions**    Peel and core the apples, then finely chop them. Peel and dice the onion and the garlic, and put them into a pan with 2–3 tbsp (30–45 ml) of cooking oil, then cook on a low heat until tender. Add the finely chopped apples and the hawthorn berries, and pour the red wine vinegar over them. Remove the herbs from any thicker stems and finely dice them, then add those to the pot as well. Simmer the mixture for 30 minutes on a gentle heat, mashing occasionally to break the skins of the hawthorn berries, then press the whole lot through the colander in batches, pushing through as much of the pulp as you can. Return the pulp to the saucepan and add brown sugar and salt to taste – usually 1 tbsp of sugar and 1 tsp of salt works well. Pour the resulting concoction into wide-necked jars and allow it to cool. This delicious ketchup is really tasty with cold meats, cheese and many other savoury dishes!

## Hawthorn elixir

**Ingredients**
- » fresh hawthorn flowering tops, gathered earlier in the year
- » hawthorn berries, gathered later on in the year
- » brandy
- » local honey

**Instructions**    This is very much a recipe of two parts: the flowers are added fresh in May, once they have opened, and then the berries are included much later on. In May, gather the best, most freshly opened flowers you can get your hands on, and pile them into a Kilner jar. No need to chop or cut these – just put them in as they are. Pour over plenty of brandy and add 1–2 tbsp (15–30 ml) of honey, then put the elixir in a dark cupboard to infuse until much later in the year. Choose a cupboard in a temperate room, not too hot but not freezing either: a kitchen cupboard or pantry works well. Stirring up the jar once or twice a week is a good idea. From September onwards, you can gather the hawthorn berries as well. Don't crush these – they are very high in pectin, which will make your elixir set solid if the skins are broken. Just gather them off the bush and pile them into the elixir whole, covering with a bit more brandy if needed, then let the whole lot infuse for another month or two. Strain out the flowers and berries and bottle the finished elixir. Take 1 tsp (5 ml) to 1 tbsp (15 ml) as a general-purpose heart tonic, to help the mind and body relax in the case of injury, or as a heart tonic for heavy hearts, sadness, times of trauma, and occasions where the heart feels bruised and melancholy. It will remind you that spring will always return and provide a bit of an open window to let the sun and fresh breezes in – very necessary when in the midst of grief or sorrow.

# Hops
## *Humulus lupulus*

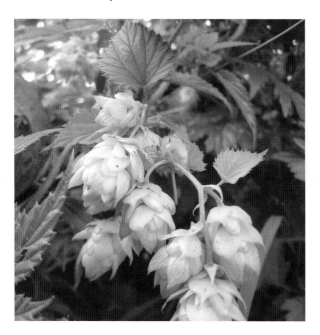

*Also known as:    beer flower*

**Family**    Cannabinaceae.

**Habitat and description**    The hop plant is a straggling, rambling, climbing perennial with lobed leaves that grow off a central, slightly rough-surfaced stem. The plant requires support and can often be found growing up trees or, if cultivated, on trellises. As most people know, hops are a primary ingredient in beer and are widely cultivated in various parts of the world; in the UK, Kent is a particularly popular area for hop growing, with hop fields and oast houses aplenty. The leaves are quite large and rich green in colour, though it is possible to get a golden version of the plant as a garden variety. The stem of the plant is very sturdy and wiry, with a faceted, slightly prickly surface. The leaves themselves are three- or five-lobed. The plants are either male or female – male hop plants have small, rather insignificant flowers, while the female plants have small cone-shaped flowers that ripen into the well-known, papery fruits from September onwards. I have often found these plants growing down by the river – rather a lovely sight when they clamber up nearby alders and twine through the plentiful brambles that also grow there – as well as scrambling merrily along train embankments and tangling through hedgerows near the local woods. The whole plant dies back over the winter and sends up fresh shoots each spring – these fresh young shoots can be eaten as an asparagus substitute and, given how many young shoots the plant can produce, will often give several yields before you need to leave the plant alone to get on with the business of growing.

**Where to find it**   Commonly growing in Europe, Western Asia and parts of North America, hops are often found in medicine gardens linked with abbeys and monasteries, as well as making a pleasing addition to the garden when trailed over arches and fences.

**Parts used**   The shoots, leaves and flowers – predominantly the dried female flowers, known as strobiles.

**When to gather**   September, when the flowers appear. If you can, twine up the stems to make a wreath or garland – this will stop the resin on the flowers from leaving a sticky residue on your baskets or drying trays.

**Medicines to make**   Teas, tinctures, elixirs; sleep pillows; creams, ointments and balms.

**Constituents**   Volatile oils; flavonoids, including chalcones such as xanthohumol, oleo-resin consisting of alpha-bitter acids including humulone and cohumulone, and beta-bitter acids including lupulene. The plant also contains tannins, phenolic acids and lipids. It contains a bitter-resin complex known as lupulin, and phyto-oestrogens, asparagin, which is responsible for the diuretic effect, choline, rutin and pectin. When the plant is dried, valeric acid is produced, which is possibly responsible for its uses in treating insomnia. Interestingly, both hops and valerian have a sedative fragrance when dried, possibly due to the presence of valeric acid.

**Planetary influence**    Mars.

**Associated deities and heroes**    Inanna, Hel, Cerridwen, Hecate, and assorted other crones and Underworld deities.

**Festival**    Samhain and Imbolc.

**Constitution**    Cold and dry.

**Actions and indications**    For anyone considering using hops, please bear in mind that if you already have trouble dealing with depression, this is not the herb for you, as it can worsen

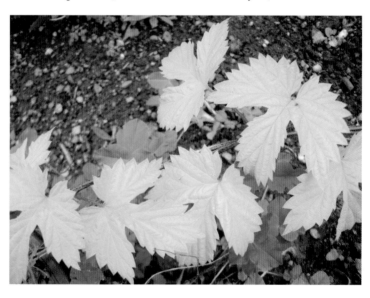

depression – another reason why beer is not recommended while struggling with low mood.

The predominant use for hops in modern herbal medicine is as a sedative for those who, for a variety of reasons, have trouble sleeping. It can also be used for restless legs, a problem that can be the bane of anyone trying to sleep. Use the plant to treat nervous anxiety, stress, hysteria and insomnia – it is particularly well suited to those folks who run hot, with a predisposition to a red complexion, red tongue, anxiety, OCD thoughts and insomnia because the brain won't switch off. Tincture is best here, in small doses of ½ tsp (2.5 ml) – it is ferociously bitter and cooling. This is one of the main herbs responsible for the "shudder and stomp" response to taking a tincture!

The plant is also used for digestive complaints, as it stimulates the production of bile, and it can therefore be used for a sluggish digestion and poor fat metabolism. Hop flowers can be used for digestive illnesses with a strong stress-related component, such as stomach ulceration and IBS, as well as ulcerative colitis, diverticulitis and nervous indigestion. They can be useful when a herb to cool excessive digestive heat is necessary. As hops are bitter, they can be used to stimulate the appetite (possibly why people drinking beer always seem to feel the need to snack on something!). Its antispasmodic properties make it useful in the treatment of spasmodic conditions of the digestive system in general.

Due to the presence of tannins, the plant can be used to stem mild diarrhoea where this is due to lax mucous membranes – particularly in the case of those who run hot. Interestingly enough, I have also used it to resolve constipation in those who run hot, with hot, dried-out mucous membranes – it moistens things back up, cools things down, and encourages normal bowel movements.

Hops contain some phyto-oestrogens and can be used to ease painful periods, to increase breast-milk production in nursing mothers, and, by extension, to calm fussy breastfed babies, if the mother takes hops medicinally. Hops can also be used to ease the transition through menopause, although, again, best avoided if you are prone to depression.

Interestingly enough, the plant depresses the libido in men but has the opposite effect on women.

As a diuretic, the plant can reduce water retention – another positive action for women who struggle with water retention associated with menstruation. It can be used to ease and relieve kidney gravel and stones, and, as a soothing diuretic, it can remove toxins from the system. It can be used in medicines aimed at relieving skin problems such as acne and eczema – possibly particularly where the skin complaint has a strong stress-related element.

A drawing ointment can be made from hops, which can be applied to boils, abscesses and bites in order to bring them to a head and promote healing. A cream of hops can be used to ward off wrinkles and keep the skin soft and supple, as well as to treat cuts and wounds, as the plant is antiseptic.

**Folklore**   The common name "hop" may derive from the Anglo-Saxon *hoppon*, meaning to climb, referring to its climbing habit.

Hops are associated with wolves and, by extension, the winter months. As a result, the plant has some connections with Brighid and the early spring festival of Imbolc. Because the plant is associated with the wolf, it also has some ties with Underworld deities.

The plant can be used to create a brown dye. According to Pliny, the Romans grew hops in their gardens and ate the young shoots as a vegetable, a practice that continues to this day. If you want to try this at home, make sure you leave enough shoots for the plant to climb with, so that you have plenty of hop flowers in the autumn.

**Dose**    Generally hops are given in tincture form to shorten the misery, as they are extremely bitter: 1:3 45% proof tincture tends to be fairly standard, but it depends on where you get it from. If you make a cottage tincture, 1 tsp (5 ml) taken no more than three times a day is fine. Smaller doses of the tincture are used for anxiety and to treat digestive complaints, and larger doses for insomnia. General dosage is up to 4 ml three times a day.

**Contraindications**    Not recommended for those who struggle with depression. If you start feeling depressed while taking hops, stop at once and see your local herbal practitioner.

# Hop recipes

## Sleep tonic blend

**Ingredients**
  » hop flowers
  » wild lettuce leaves
  » lemon balm leaves
  » German chamomile flowers
  » vodka or brandy – as strong as you can get

**Instructions**    As with many of the elixirs, this is a recipe where ingredients will need to be added as and when they come ready. Start off with the wild lettuce, lemon balm and chamomile, adding them to a jar when they are at their best. The flowers can be added whole, but the leaves will need to be finely chopped or shredded. Cover with plenty of alcohol, and leave the whole lot to steep.

Later in the year, you can add the hop flowers. These need to be gathered at the peak of their development, just as they turn papery, and they will leave a strongly scented resin on your fingers after gathering. Just bring a couple of handfuls into the kitchen, shred them and put them into the tonic blend, pop the lid on, and make sure you shake the jar every other day for a few weeks. Eventually you can strain out the herbs and bottle the tonic. Take 1 tsp (5 ml) an hour before bed to encourage the mind to wind down and to help you get a restful night's sleep.

## Hop and lavender sleep pillow

**Ingredients / equipment**
- » a few handfuls of dried hop flowers
- » 2 tbsp of dried lavender flowers
- » cotton fabric with a pretty print on it
- » needle and thread

**Instructions**   Cut a rectangle of fabric, aiming for around 35 cm (14 in.) on the long side and around 25 cm (10 in.) on the short side. Fold the fabric in half with the pattern facing inwards and sew around one long side and one short side to create a pouch. You can use a sewing machine for this if you have one: it will give a much tighter stitch – or you can sew it by hand, using running stitch or back stitch, but keep the stitches small and close together if you can, so the herbs don't escape. Turn the pouch the right way out, using a needle hooked into the corners to gently winkle them out properly, then stuff in a few good handfuls of hop flowers and the lavender flowers. Turn the two open edges inwards by around 0.5 cm, then stitch along the top to close the pouch. This can be slotted into your pillowcase with the pillow or tucked underneath it – just refresh the scent as needed with drops of essential oil once or twice a year. You can also replace the ingredients entirely every year if you want to, making it a lovely autumn ritual to be completed.

## Hop and marshmallow leaf drawing ointment

**Ingredients**
- » several handfuls of fresh hop flowers
- » an equal amount of fresh or dried marshmallow leaves
- » organic vegetable or seed oil
- » beeswax

**Instructions**    Pile the shredded, clean and surface-dry herbs into the top of a double boiler and pour over enough oil to cover, then let the whole lot infuse on a moderate heat for at least half an hour, preferably longer. I do recommend double infusing if you can, so once the oil has changed colour, filter out the first batch of herbs and replace them with a second batch. Steep again for another hour, then strain out the herbs. Add 18 g of beeswax per 100 ml (3½ fl oz) of oil and return it to the hob, stirring until the wax has melted; then pour the resulting ointment into wide-necked jars. To use the ointment, simply scrape out a small amount, depending on the size of the area you are trying to draw detritus or pus out of. Smear it onto a clean plaster or piece of cloth or bandage and place it carefully over the target area, using sticky plasters to fasten it in place if you need to. If you are allergic to plasters, you may need to bandage it in place instead. Leave this in place for at least half a day if you can. This will encourage boils or abscesses to come to a head and drain cleanly, after which they can be treated with calendula to clean them thoroughly and encourage them to heal. This ointment can also be used to draw grit out of grazes or cuts – as above, douse the wound with calendula once you are sure it is clean. This will sting, but it will encourage it to heal clean and fast.

# Horse chestnut
## *Aesculus hippocastanum*

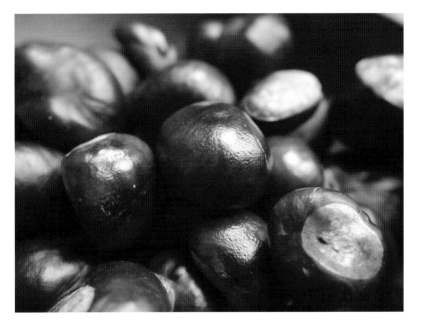

*Also known as:*    conker

**Family**    Sapindaceae.

**Habitat and description**    The tall and stately horse chestnut is not actually indigenous to this country – it was imported from Asia in the sixteenth century, in order to be planted in fashionable gardens. Over time it has naturalised in the UK and now self-seeds readily from the glossy chestnut-coloured conkers, sprouting up quite happily in hedgerows, woods and other areas. The tree tends to form extremely tall, straight columns, branching at the top, with greyish green-coloured bark which is usually fairly smooth to the touch. Buds form on the tree in the autumn and winter and are covered in a protective gum that stops the frost from nipping them. They are some of the first to begin to stretch open in the spring. Conversely, the tree is also one of the first to turn russet and drop its leaves in the autumn. The leaves, once they unfurl in spring, form in groups of five to seven on one stem and are a shape similar to that of a peacock's feather, spreading palmate with light toothing around the edges. The flowers, which open from May to June, are ivory with pink centres, forming in tall spikes on the branches. These give way to the familiar horse chestnuts, which ripen slowly and finally open in September and October.

**Where to find it**   Gardens, hedgerows and woodlands in the UK, parts of Asia and Europe, and also parts of the USA and Canada.

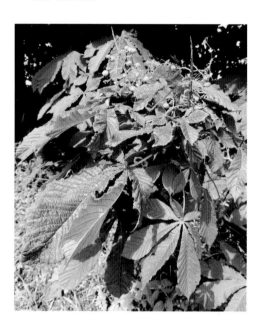

**Parts used**   The horse chestnuts, leaves and bark.

**When to gather**   Horse chestnuts in autumn. Leaves in summer, and bark year round. Flowers in late spring and summer.

**Medicines to make**   Decoctions and infusions; liniments and tinctures; baths and washes. Never to be taken internally except under the guidance of a professional herbalist.

**Constituents**   Triterpenoid saponins including escin and tannins; quinines; sterols; fatty acids including linolenic acid; flavonoid glycosides and coumarins.

**Planetary influence**   Jupiter.

**Associated deities and heroes**   Flower deities, including Blodeuwedd.

**Festival**   Beltane.

**Constitution**   Warm and dry.

**Actions and indications**   Traditionally horse chestnut, made into a gel or salve, is used topically as a strong astringent for varicose veins and piles. A decoction or infusion can be made and used topically for ulcers, either as a bath or applied as a spray using a spray bottle, depending on the level of discomfort in the patient.

Horse chestnut makes an excellent salve for cuts, grazes and ringworm, again due to the tannins present, and can also be used as part of a cream recipe to reduce the appearance of cellulite. A bath of the chestnuts or plaister of the ointment can be used to relieve prolapsed discs, tightening and toning the connective tissues and encouraging them to sit back in their correct place. Combine horse chestnut with woodruff and wintergreen for chilblains as a cream or salve, or even use it as a warm hand bath.

Internally, the tincture or decoction can be used very carefully in drop doses for venous health, including poor circulation, venous insufficiency and valve prolapse, but this should only be done under the guidance of a professional herbalist. It can also be of benefit in cases of passive venous congestion, where the heart has to work harder to shift blood around the body, leading to high blood pressure. Lower-limb oedema and heavy legs, as well as swollen ankles, can also benefit from the herb internally (again under professional guidance): consider using a bath of it externally as well in this case to really tackle the problem from both sides.

One of the best-known uses of horse chestnut is in the treatment of varicose veins and haemorrhoids – it is used topically as well as internally, as drop doses of weak tincture in water when taken as a medicine. A strong tea can be used for acne and rosacea of the face, as it acts as an astringent and tonic to the blood vessels – again, if rosacea is the issue, consider also taking drop doses internally to tone the blood vessels (but only under the guidance of a professional herbalist). Drop doses can also be useful in the case of OCD with insomnia, piles and venous congestion, where a bounding, wiry pulse is present.

The flowers can be used as a bath for calming and settling the nerves.

**Folklore**    The conker has been used as a playground game for generations. Conkers are gathered, drilled and suspended on a shoelace, and groups of children form pairs and try to hit each other's conkers using their own suspended weapons. The victor is the one with the conker undamaged after their partner's has succumbed to the casual violence on show.

Traditionally, carrying conkers in the pocket has been linked with good luck and wealth; depending on the folklore of the region, one or three conkers should be carried. In the US, carrying conkers was said to boost a man's virility.

Having conkers in the house has long been used as a way to deter spiders, the conkers tucked into the nooks and crannies that spiders like to set up house in. Replace the conkers every year to keep spiders at bay.

**Dose**    Go for a weak tincture of 1:10 30%, or see your local herbalist to obtain a suitable tincture plus instructions. I tend to recommend a maximum of 2 tsp (10 ml) of tincture in a week's dose of medicine, especially to begin with, and between 5 and 20 drops twice a day for venous issues and haemorrhoids if used as a single remedy – traditionally given in a little water. If you are using it internally (with professional guidance), consider combining it with other herbs for the circulatory system.

**Contraindications**    Avoid during pregnancy and breastfeeding. Internal use is not recommended without professional guidance – this herb can make you very sick in larger doses, in part due to the presence of saponins, which create plenty of foam if you shake the chestnuts up in alcohol or water but which also cause severe nausea.

# Horse chestnut recipes

## Horse chestnut and herb robert salve for piles and varicose veins

**Ingredients**
- » 1 pint of loosely packed horse chestnut leaves
- » 1 pint of herb robert leaves and flowers
- » organic seed oil
- » beeswax

**Instructions**    Finely chop the leaves and flowers as thoroughly as possible and put them into the top of a double boiler, covering with the oil until a depth of just shy of one finger's width of oil is on top of the plant matter. Simmer the water in the lower pan gently until the oil has turned a deep, rich green, then filter out the plant matter. Add 12 g of beeswax for every 100 ml (3½ fl oz) of oil and return the oil and wax to the pan, bringing to a gentle simmer until the wax has melted. Stir thoroughly and pour into jars.

This salve is strongly astringent and can be used topically for piles and varicose veins. You can add lavender essential oil if preferred; however, as the salve is likely to be used on sensitive areas, I tend not to add fragrance to it.

## Horse chestnut liniment

**Ingredients**
- » plenty of fresh horse chestnuts
- » vodka

**Instructions**    This is very simple to make! Just pack the horse chestnuts into a sturdy bag and bash the bag thoroughly with a rolling pin to really break down the nuts: this is very therapeutic if you are stressed out. Pack the fragments into a Kilner jar and pour over enough vodka to cover them, plus a good couple of centimetres on top. Put the lid on and let it steep for at least two weeks, then strain out the plant matter through two layers of muslin, and then through a coffee filter paper. You can apply this liniment topically to the legs to encourage varicose veins to shrink, and also use it in drop doses internally (under professional guidance) to act as a venous astringent.

## Horse chestnut plaister for prolapsed discs

**Ingredients**
- » fresh horse chestnuts
- » organic seed oil
- » beeswax

**Instructions**   This is a delightfully fun recipe to make, mostly due to the violence with which you need to bash the horse chestnuts before infusing in oil! I recommend piling them into a clean pillow case or cloth bag, closing the top, and either jumping up and down on them or using a rolling pin to beat them into smallish pieces. Once you are happy that you have broken them down sufficiently, pile them into the top of a double boiler or a slow cooker kept just for the purpose, pour over plenty of oil with an extra centimetre on top, and give the mixture a long, slow infusion for at least an hour – longer if possible. Once the conkers have fully infused, strain the resulting horse chestnut oil through kitchen roll and add 16 g of beeswax per 100 ml (3½ fl oz) of oil. Return the mixture to the double boiler, warm through and stir until the wax has melted, then pour the mixture onto clean squares of cloth placed on dinner plates. Let the mixture set, peel the cloths off the plates, and put them onto large squares of grease-proof paper. Scrape off any ointment left behind and smear that onto the cloths as well, then fold the paper over and roll them up. Store the plaisters in glass jars, complete with label and instructions. To use, unroll them and apply them gently to the area in question, bandaging lightly in place to keep the ointment where it needs to be. Leave it in place for at least an hour, longer if possible, to tighten the ligaments and tendons around the area and encourage the disc back into its proper place.

# Horseradish
## *Armoracia rusticana*

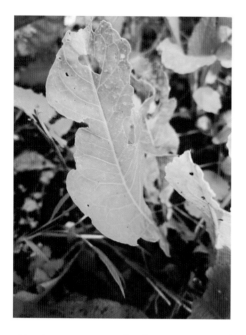

*Also known as:*    red cole, mountain radish, great raifort

**Family**    Brassicaceae.

**Habitat and description**    Cultivated by many vegetable grow-
ers for its pungent root, horseradish can also be found growing
wild in verges and hedgerows. I have seen many clusters of
it growing across my native county of Lincolnshire, where
it can be found in great swathes across the edges of fields,
becoming somewhat of a nuisance. Horseradish leaves look
a little like those of the common dock, but, on the whole,
are slightly larger and thicker and lightly toothed. They are

also more of a blue-green colour, whereas those of dock are more yellow-green. In the summer, horseradish produces tall spikes of small white flowers, like many other members of the same plant family. It thrives in good, fertile soil, where it will grow up to a metre (3¼ ft) tall, and it can be easily grown in the garden, provided it has the right ground to grow in. The root is substantial and cone shaped, and the whole plant can regrow easily from a tiny piece of the root left behind when harvesting.

The root, once harvested, needs to be prepared fairly quickly and is almost always used fresh – once dried, the root has none of the exciting odour that emerges from the fresh cut plant. Older roots become more bitter than pungent. Sinus-rippingly strong, the evaporating volatile oils of the grated or chopped fresh root can cause real discomfort to the eyes.

**Where to find it**    Britain and Europe, from the Mediterranean all the way across to Scandinavia; also North America.

**Parts used**    The root and occasionally the leaves.

**When to gather**    Autumn and winter.

**Medicines to make**    Tinctures, vinegars and honegars, infused honey, liniments, syrups. It makes a surprisingly tasty elixir.

**Constituents**    Volatile oils, resins and vitamin C; glucosinolates, including sinigrin; and horseradish peroxidase, which is being investigated for anti-cancer properties.

**Planetary influence**    Mars.

**Associated deities and heroes**    None known at present, but a case could be made for deities associated with fire, such as Thor and Thunor.

**Festival**    Mabon.

**Constitution**    Hot and dry.

**Actions and indications**    Horseradish is predominantly known as a cardiovascular stimulant, boosting sluggish circulation, and also has rubefacient properties when applied to the skin, where the irritant properties of the volatile oils draw blood to the area of application.

It can be used both topically and internally as an expectorant, and the antibacterial properties make it particularly useful for congested, infected chest conditions where large amounts of phlegm are produced that the body is unable to remove through coughing. Taken internally and applied externally to the chest, the back, and the soles of the feet, horseradish can help the body to thin and remove excess phlegm. As a fiery, heating herb, it also makes an excellent remedy to take at the onset of coughs, colds and influenza, again because of its antibacterial properties, circulatory tonic action and general heat levels, which relieve the discomfort of flu. The root has diaphoretic properties, meaning that when drunk hot, it can encourage the body to have a good sweat, lowering the body's temperature and breaking fevers. Some recipes for Fire Cider Vinegar feature the use of horseradish.

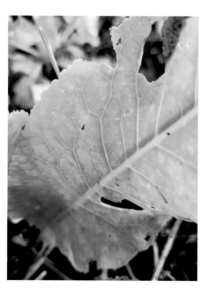

Another use is as a strong diuretic, and as a result of this it has a long history of use for the treatment of dropsy. It makes a useful remedy for oedema coupled with lax tissues and a cold digestion, kicking the body back into action.

Topically it can be a useful salve or liniment for the relief of Raynaud's disease and chilblains, where it combines well with a range of other herbs. In addition, it can be used as a poultice, balm, liniment or plaister for rheumatic and musculoskeletal pain; traditionally the fresh, grated or chopped root was used and was left in place until a blister formed. The root has a long reputation in the curing of severe joint pain due to its ability to pull blood to the area and improve overall joint health. If you want to apply horseradish topically, make sure you place a cloth between the root and your skin.

Traditionally it has been eaten all over the world as a condiment, particularly coupled with fish and red meat. This is for more than just the flavour – the herb is also a useful liver, gallbladder and pancreas stimulant and is well suited to cold, stagnant digestive systems prone to producing a lot of phlegm, particularly those where rich foods cause long-lasting, grinding nausea and a tendency to fatty liver. The bitter properties of the root can boost a flagging appetite, very useful for the elderly and those with poor interest in food for a variety of reasons. Avoid use during pregnancy, though.

**Folklore**   Horseradish was apparently named after its use as an animal feed – slightly erroneously, as unfortunately it was responsible for the death of a number of animals that had eaten too much of it: the furiously martial nature of the plant causes massive inflammation of the digestive tract and is one of the main reasons why we use it only in small doses.

The Greek oracles at Delphi were of the opinion that horseradish was worth its weight in gold – a sentiment that can be agreed with, crossing, as it does, the boundary between medicine and food.

**Dose**    Small doses of the tincture or drop doses are recommended to begin with, as larger doses can cause nausea and vomiting. Start with 5 drops and work up from there, as needed.

**Contraindications**    Avoid during pregnancy. Best suited to deeply entrenched, cold, phlegm-producing conditions. As with many brassicas, use with caution or avoid completely in cases of an underactive thyroid. Avoid in overheated conditions, where a hectic complexion and red tongue are present.

# Horseradish recipes

## Horseradish honey or elixir

**Ingredients**
- » fresh horseradish root
- » local runny honey
- » alcohol – brandy or vodka, as preferred

**Instructions**    Thoroughly scrub the fresh root once you've unearthed it, then roll it vigorously in a clean tea towel to take off any excess moisture clinging to the surface. Grate the root on the finest grater setting and stir it into a jar of honey – 2 tbsp of root to one 350 ml jar of honey tends to work quite well, but you can make this as strong as you want it. This can be left to infuse for as long as you want, and then you can either strain out the grated root or leave it in and add it to cups of tea or cook with it as is. The honey can be added to a traditional cough, cold and flu tea of mint, yarrow and elder as an extra way to relieve the discomfort of coughs and colds, or taken to boost the digestion. Alternatively, steep the grated root in brandy or vodka and add the honey to this mixture. Either makes a tasty concoction.

## Horseradish chilblain balm

**Ingredients**
- » fresh horseradish root
- » organic seed oil
- » horse chestnut oil (see Horse chestnut for instructions as part of the plaister recipe)
- » beeswax
- » rosemary and wintergreen essential oils

**Instructions**    Scrub and surface-dry the root as much as you can, then grate it on the larger setting. Once grated, put the root into a dehydrator on the lower setting to evaporate off some of the excess water or, alternatively, spread the grated or chopped root in a thin layer on a baking sheet and pop it into a low oven with the door ajar. Make sure you don't completely dry the root out, though, as doing so will mean loss of a lot of the pungent oils that make it so helpful. Once the root is still flexible but not soggy, pile it into a slow cooker and pour over enough seed oil to cover it. Let the whole thing infuse on a low setting overnight, until the oil is pungent, then strain out the spent root, which can be composted.

Measure out 50 ml (1¾ fl oz) of this oil and add an equal amount of horse chestnut infused oil to make 100 ml (3½ fl oz) of the combined oil, then add 12 g of beeswax per 100 ml of the oil mixture. Put the ingredients into a double boiler over a moderate heat and warm through until the wax has melted, then stir it thoroughly. Add 5 drops each of the two essential oils, stir again, and pour the concoction into jars. This can be used for chilblains as well as for sore joints and muscles and will pull blood to the area. You can also make a version without the horse chestnut, using mint and rosemary oils, which can be applied sparingly to the sinuses to relieve sinusitis – be careful, though, because horseradish in the eyes can cause significant pain! You can also use this as a chest rub in the case of infected chest conditions where a lot of phlegm has been produced that won't move.

## Horseradish tincture or vinegar

**Ingredients**
» fresh horseradish root
» vodka or unpasteurised cider vinegar

**Instructions**    As above, scrub and roughly dry the surface of the root, then either grate it or use a sharp knife to slice it into thin discs. The prepared root can then be piled into a clean jar and the alcohol or vinegar poured over the top, allowing several centimetres of liquid on top of the roots. Leave the root to infuse in the liquid for a month, then strain out the herbs and bottle the resulting concoction. Take a 1 tsp (5 ml) dose of the tincture or vinegar to boost a sluggish digestive tract that struggles to cope with fatty or rich foods. The tincture or vinegar can also be used as a liniment on cold, sore muscles or arthritic joints, or on the chest as a rub in the case of phlegmy chest infections, where the phlegm is stuck and won't move properly.

You can also make this recipe including fresh sliced elecampane root and plenty of fresh root ginger – just use equal proportions of each, infuse them in the vinegar for several weeks, and then strain them out. Take 1 tsp (5 ml) in hot water at the onset of a cold to really kick-start the healing process.

# Horsetail

*Equisetum arvense*

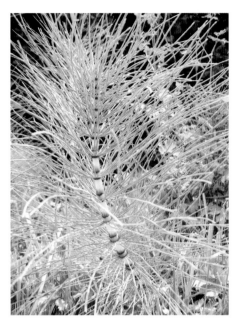

*Also known as:* shave-grass, bottle-brush, paddock pipes, pewterwort, Dutch rushes

**Family**  Equisetaceae.

**Habitat and description**  Anyone who has had horsetail in their garden will have reason to curse it roundly, as it is almost impossible to get rid of! It is, however, one of the oldest plants in the world, and it does have a goodly array of useful properties and medicines that can be made from it – not to mention the sheer awesomeness of being in the presence of a plant that dates back so far. Horsetail bears a slight resemblance to ephedra, a plant not native to this country. The stems grow upwards from creeping rhizomes, which help it to spread over large areas of ground. Two kinds of stems are produced – fertile, and barren. Both stems are hollow, jointed, brittle, erect and grooved in appearance, with no leaves – instead, long slender lobes that look a little like long pine needles are produced in a whorl around the stem, making the whole plant look rather like a bottle brush. The fertile stems are unbranched and wither in the spring, producing spores with which the plant reproduces, much like the ferns. It likes growing in damp places, and it accumulates large quantities of silica in its stems.

**Where to find it**    Horsetail is native to pretty much the entire northern hemisphere, including the arctic regions.

**Parts used**    Green shoots of the barren stems, which are gathered in the summer, long after the fertile stems have died back.

**When to gather**    Late summer.

**Medicines to make**    Powder, capsules, infused oil, tincture (both fresh and dried), plant ashes.

**Constituents**    Alkaloids, including nicotine and palustrine;

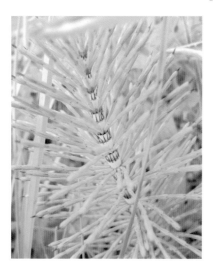

flavonoids, such as apigenin and quercetin glycosides; sterols; silicic acids; caffeic acid.

**Planetary influence**    Saturn.

**Associated deities and heroes**    None known at present, but possibly Pluto, Hades and related Underworld deities. There are grounds to link it with the Ancestors, as well.

**Festival**    Samhain, given its links with the past.

**Constitution**    Cold and dry.

**Actions and indications**    Horsetail has a decent array of medicinal uses. Its strongly astringent action makes it handy for bleeding and haemorrhage. It is also used to encourage better connective tissue health, especially where disc prolapse, repeatedly torn or pulled ligaments, or over-relaxed ligaments are present – it can be used internally and externally for these issues. If using it internally, go for drop doses of tincture: you are aiming to remind the connective tissue how to work and to give the body the lesson of where and how internal boundaries need to operate, and for this you don't need huge doses – nor are they advised, as in large doses the silica content irritates the body.

Horsetail has an affinity with the bladder and kidneys, making it a soothing and non-irritating diuretic remedy suitable for relieving cystitis, prostatitis and nephritis. It also has some antispasmodic properties and can be used for incontinence, blood in the urine and bedwetting as the antispasmodic, astringent properties tighten and tone over-relaxed valves and mucous membranes.

It has been used as an immune enhancer, as it stimulates the production of white blood cells, so use it with caution and consult your doctor if you are taking immune-suppressing drugs.

It can be combined with calcium as a bone-density tonic – perhaps consider nettle and horsetail decoction three or four times a week to really encourage good bone health. This blend can also be used to strengthen hair and nails, and as a hair rinse to relieve dandruff and oily hair.

In the past, horsetail was used to encourage tissue repair in the lungs after tuberculosis infection, and it encourages better resistance to the bacteria that cause it.

It combines very well with pasque flower and rose for inhibiting uterine fibroids, and it can be helpful in slowing regrowth after some have been removed. A strong decoction of horsetail is an emmenagogue and should be avoided during pregnancy.

Previously the plant ashes were used for acid-stomach issues, as they contain high levels of silica – up to 75% in some cases.

A strong decoction or tincture of horsetail is antifungal, and it can be used to treat fungal toenails where the fungus is growing under the toenail. I suggest making a footbath out of it for this purpose and then following the footbath with an application of the tincture as well.

It is considered best to pick horsetail that grows in full sunlight, not that which grows in the shade. It needs to be tinctured or decocted fresh – it is hard to dry the herb, as water tends to accumulate in all of the little joints. Be careful when you gather it – make sure there is no brown spotting on the leaves or stem, as this is a fungal growth.

**Folklore**    Horsetail is one of the few plants from the time of the dinosaurs, with fossilised remains of the plant's relatives having been dated back to the Carboniferous era.

**Dose**    I recommend 10–25 drops three times a day. Too much of it won't sit well, as it is just too much "sand" for the body.

**Contraindications**    Horsetail can cause contact dermatitis in some people. Avoid during pregnancy.

# Horsetail recipes

## Horsetail and nettle decoction

**Ingredients**
- » a couple of decent-sized handfuls of fresh horsetail, gathered in late summer from sunny spots
- » a few tablespoons (up to 50 g) of dried nettle tops, harvested between March and early May
- » 570 ml (20 fl oz) of water

**Instructions**    There are two methods for making a decoction – short and long – and both are described briefly here.

To make a short decoction, finely chop or shred the horsetail (you will find kitchen scissors helpful here) and pile it into a pan with the dried nettle tops. (If you had cut back your nettles earlier in the year, you may find fresh growth coming through from September onwards, and if this is the case, you can instead use this fresh plant growth in your decoction.) Pour 570 ml (20 fl oz) of water over the herbs and bring to a gentle simmer for 10 minutes, until the water has decreased by about a third. Take the pan off the heat and filter out the herbs. Take 1 tbsp (15 ml) doses three times a day to boost mineral levels in the body, to act as a gentle diuretic and tonic for the kidneys and bladder, and to improve connective tissue health. Short decoctions can keep for up to three days in the fridge.

To make a long decoction, you will need to keep simmering the herbs on the hob for several hours, topping up the water periodically. This long, slow method for infusing the herbs in the water will result in a much stronger, more stable decoction that can be kept for much longer in the fridge. As it is a stronger medicine, take half of the dose given for the short decoction. Either decoction can be used as an antifungal footbath if needed.

## Horsetail and nettle hair rinse for dark or red hair

**Ingredients**
- » 570 ml (20 fl oz) of the horsetail and nettle short decoction made in the previous recipe, or 285 ml (10 fl oz) of the long decoction
- » 200 ml (7 fl oz) of cider vinegar
- » rosemary essential oil

**Instructions**   Mix up all the ingredients in a bottle and add up to 10 drops of essential oil, shaking it up thoroughly to disperse the oil through the liquid. Use this as a hair rinse to bring lustre and shine to the hair, to balance hair oils and to relieve dandruff. Best suited to dark or red hair.

## Horsetail tincture

**Ingredients**
- » 1 pint or more of fresh horsetail tops, gathered in late summer or early autumn
- » vodka – as strong as you can get

**Instructions**   Finely chop the fresh horsetail tops using scissors and pile them into a clean Kilner jar, then pour over the alcohol. Let the whole lot infuse for at least a month, then strain out the herbs and bottle the resulting tincture. Go for drop doses if possible – up to 30 drops twice a day to ease connective tissue disorders and act as an astringent tonic for the body. You can also apply this neat to fungal toenails.

# Ivy
## *Hedera helix*

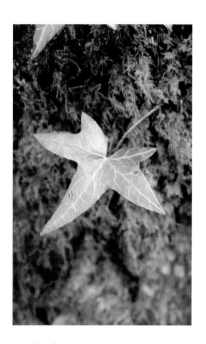 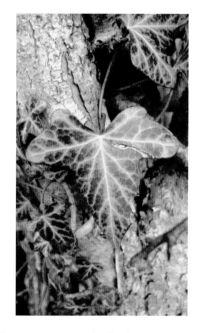

*Also known as:* cat's foot, me hoofe, robin-run-in-the-hedge, true ivy, tun-hoof, common ivy

**Family**   Araliaceae.

**Habitat and description**   Ivy is a familiar sight around the British Isles, with its deep-green leaves with up to five points and creamy or pale-green veins. The leaves usually grow in roughly opposing pairs on long, trailing stems, with thread-like aerial roots growing on the undersides – these allow the plant to climb up walls and tree trunks. The leaves are quite leathery, shiny, and paler coloured on the underside. The berries are small, beginning bright green and, over time, turning purplish-black in colour and forming in round clusters.

Ivy will grow in most places and will often twine around trees and up walls, finding a footing in the most unwelcoming crevices. Once ivy has found a home in the garden, it is very difficult to eradicate, as the smallest stem with a bit of root on it will re-establish an ivy "colony". The plant is parasitic and has been known to kill trees by twining around them too thickly.

**Where to find it**    Most of Europe, as well as parts of Western Asia.

**Parts used**    Leaves. The berries are poisonous and should not be taken internally; they can, though, be used to make a green dye for fabric.

**When to gather**    Leaves, pretty much year-round; berries for dye-making only, when black.

**Medicines to make**    Tinctures; infused oils and balms; poultices; tea infusions; washes and skin baths; powders.

**Constituents**    The plant contains antimutagenic saponins based on oleanolic acid, as well as sterols; polyacetylenes such as falcarinol, which can sometimes be responsible for causing allergic reactions; essential oils; flavonoids, including rutin; and caffeic-acid derivatives, including rosmarinic acid. The saponins and sapogenins are the primary active ingredients, responsible for the expectorant, amoebicidal, antifungal and molluscicidal properties of the plant.

**Planetary influence**    Saturn (unsurprisingly).

**Associated deities and heroes**    Arianrhod, Cerridwen, Isis, Osiris, Persephone, Kore, Saturn, The White Goddess.

**Festival**    All, and none. Perhaps most specifically Beltane, Yule, Imbolc and Lammas.

**Constitution**    Cold and dry (fitting, as this is a herb of Saturn).

**Actions and indications**   Although ivy is not commonly used in current herbal medicine, it has been used for a variety of purposes in the past.

The fresh young leaves are primarily used, and these are generally harvested between August and September, though I have used the young leaves pretty much all year round. The bark was previously used for sores caused by syphilis, though the berries are equally effective – however, they are toxic and purgative and have been known in the past to cause fatalities. Ivy is analgesic and antispasmodic. Topically, it can be used to treat neuralgia and related nerve disorders, rheumatic pain and cellulitis, although the fresh leaves have been known to cause contact dermatitis. Internally, the herb can be used (with caution) to treat whooping cough. It is generally antispasmodic and gently sedative.

Ivy has been widely used to treat bronchitis and catarrh as an expectorant, though I don't recommend it for home use, as it is very strong. It is especially efficacious in the treatment of chronic bronchitis, bringing about improved expectoration of phlegm and reduced levels of pain. The primary active ingredients in the plant are the saponins and sapogenins, the latter in high levels. Extracts of ivy leaf are often used in preparations for the topical treatment of cellulite – with some success, although few clinical trials have been carried out to support this use.

A poultice of the fresh leaves can be used to treat leg ulcers and nerve complaints, as well as raised glands in the neck. A good, strong balm of it can be used for arthritis and rheumatic pain, neuralgia, and inflamed lymph nodes. A wash made using a tea of the leaves can be used to relieve sunburn and eczema. The powder of the plant, made from its leaves, can be inhaled to treat nasal polyps.

Many of the plants belonging to the Araliaceae family seem to have some form of adaptogenic and tonic action.

The plant seems to be cool and drying in action, with a sweet flavour, and may be of benefit with damp, stagnant conditions (defined as kapha, according to the Ayurvedic system, but which could be considered as phlegmatic in the Western tradition). This would certainly explain why the plant is used to treat many stagnant conditions, although it may only be cooling to the first degree rather than to the third or fourth degree. If you want to work with it at home, use it with extreme caution, as this is a powerful herb.

**Folklore**    Ivy has a large body of folklore. It is often connected to the vine in myth and legend, with both having the ability to change the consciousness – the ivy has, rightly or wrongly, gained a reputation for being able to undo drunkenness, and it can often be seen to this effect on inn signs. The chewing of ivy leaves (which, however, are poisonous) may induce a temporary alteration of mental state, facilitating inward journeys.

The Greek gods Dionysus and Ariadne are associated with the ivy plant, as are Dionysus's followers, the Bassairds. The ivy has a longstanding association with rebirth and immortality, as it is evergreen. The religious cult of women who followed Bacchus / Dionysus were known as the Bacchae, and, after drinking a mixture of fermented ivy, fly agaric and pine sap, they rampaged around the countryside, tearing animals and humans to pieces. Ivy represents the cycles of the moon and has a strong link to fertility and the menstrual cycle as a result of this connection.

Ivy has a longstanding two-faced reputation, both good and bad, as it is associated with the Goddess and therefore partakes of the entwined principles of life and death. The plant was classically associated with desolation and melancholia in eighteenth-century England and is, as a result, often found growing around picturesque ruins.

**Dose**    2 ml per day of a 1:10 leaf tincture in 25% alcohol. A maceration in vinegar can be used topically and as a mouth wash. As mentioned earlier, use this plant with caution, as it is rather strong!

**Contraindications** The berries are poisonous and should never be used. The plant can cause contact dermatitis in some people. As already mentioned, this is a very strong plant and is not recommended for home use internally except under the guidance of a medical herbalist.

# Ivy recipes

## Ivy balm

**Ingredients**
- » 2–3 handfuls of freshly picked ivy leaves, picked on a dry day
- » organic sunflower oil
- » beeswax
- » essential oil: mint works well, as does ravensara, which has a specific action on the nerves

**Instructions** Check the leaves carefully for any bugs, then finely shred them using a mezzaluna or a sharp knife. (Make sure you wash your hands thoroughly once you have finished chopping the leaves – ivy can be poisonous even in relatively small doses. I'd also recommend using a chopping board that is kept just for preparing this medicine.) Pile them into the top of a clean, dry double boiler and pour over enough oil to cover the shredded leaves, then warm gently until the water in the bottom of the double boiler simmers.

Keep the double boiler simmering until the oil has changed colour and become a rich green. You can do this part on the top of a wood-burning stove, if you have one. Once the oil has turned green, strain out the herbs and return the oil to the top of the double boiler. Add 12 g of beeswax per 100 ml

(3½ fl oz) of oil, and warm again, stirring the mixture until the wax has melted. Add 25 drops of your chosen essential oil per 100 ml (3½ fl oz) of oil, stir briefly, and pour the mixture into jars. Allow to cool and put the lid on, then label it well. This balm is wonderful for nerve issues, including neuralgia and trapped nerves, and it can also be used for rheumatism and arthritis.

## Ivy leaf skin wash

**Ingredients**
- » ½ pint, loosely packed, of ivy leaves
- » 570 ml (20 fl oz) of water

**Instructions**    Finely chop the leaves and pop them into a pan used only for medicine making. Pour over the water, and put the whole thing onto a moderate heat to simmer for 10 minutes, then turn off the heat. Let the decoction cool, and use it as a skin wash for sunburn and eczema.

# Marshmallow / Mallow
## *Althaea officinalis / Malva*

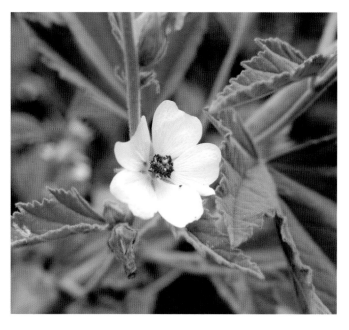

*Also known as:* high mallow, mauls, cheese flower, blue mallow, common mallow, mallards, schloss tea, cheeses, mortification root

**Family**   Malvaceae: Marshmallow (*Althaea officinalis*); common mallow (*Malva sylvestris*); musk mallow (*Malva moschata*).

**Habitat and description**   Marshmallow is a tall-growing perennial often cultivated in gardens for its attractive silvery-grey, velvety, roughly spearhead-shaped foliage and tall stems of pale pinky-lilac flowers. Common mallow is a rather pretty perennial that grows to about 1 m (3 ft) tall. It is a regular denizen of hedgerows and roadsides (including near where

I live) and can even be found tucking itself in by rivers and streams. The leaves are lobed and dark green in colour, with fine toothing and an interesting frilly shape a little like Lady's mantle. The flowers are dark pink-purple and slightly stripy and grow in clusters on the stems. Musk mallow has pale pink or creamy white flowers, and paler green leaves that are much more deeply toothed. It is another perennial, growing to around 0.75 m (2 ft) tall; like common mallow, it enjoys growing along roadsides and in hedgerows, especially in places where it gets plenty of sun.

**Where to find it**   The UK, Europe and parts of Asia; parts of Africa, Egypt and more temperate zones, like North America.

**Parts used**   The flowers, leaves, root and whole plant.

**When to gather**   Root in late autumn and early winter; flowers and leaves when the whole plant is in flower.

**Medicines to make**   Cold infusions; hot infusions and decoctions; tinctures; salves; poultices for drawing grit out of

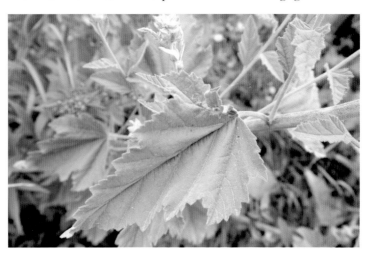

wounds and encouraging boils to come to a head and drain; herb-infused honey.

**Constituents**   Starch, plenty of mucilage, pectin, flavonoids, tannins, scopoletin, oil, sugars, asparagine, cellulose. The roots contain a large amount of mucilage, as well as polysaccharides, flavonoids, coumarins and polyphenolic acids including caffeic, salicylic and vanillic acids. The leaf contains mucilages, flavonoids and polyphenolics, such as caffeic acid, which is also to be found in the flower.

**Planetary influence**   Venus / the Moon.

**Associated deities and heroes**   Osiris, Althea, Venus, Aphrodite, Shiva; probably also other cultural representations of Venus, including deities such as Inanna, who, despite having a considerably darker side to her than is generally conceded to a face of the Goddess of Love, is nevertheless often seen as the Sumerian counterpart of Venus. You could probably also include Freya in this list as well, for similar reasons.

**Festival**   Beltane.

**Constitution**   Cool and moist – the whole plant is gently demulcent, softening and moistening.

**Actions and indications**   These members of the Malvaceae family – marshmallow, common mallow, and musk mallow – can be used pretty much interchangeably. The primary use for marshmallow and its relatives is as a soothing demulcent, suitable for many inflamed conditions afflicting the mucous membranes of the urinary tract, respiratory tract and digestive system. All members of the family can be used to soothe ulceration of the digestive system and related digestive upsets like gastritis, peptic ulceration and inflammation of the system in general, such as that caused by IBS, IBD and ulcerative colitis. They bring relief to mild constipation as well as to diarrhoea.

They are a wonderful expectorant and demulcent and can be used to ease catarrh, dry coughs and related bronchial complaints, such as bronchitis. They make a useful mild antitussive to soothe coughs in general, as well as to ease laryngitis and pneumonia, making it a lovely addition to cough syrups.

As a soothing demulcent for the urinary tract, they can be used to ease cystitis and related urinary-tract infections, as well as nephritis and urinary calculi. They can also be used to give relief to those who suffer from high blood pressure with related water retention. The leaf is the part most often used to treat urinary-tract problems as well as respiratory-tract issues. The root is most often used to treat digestive-tract ailments, having a much higher mucilage content – indeed, marshmallow root tincture often has a delightfully thick, syrupy consistency to it.

The root can also have a lubricating effect on the joints and skeleton in general, which makes these plants useful back-up herbs in the treatment of arthritis and related joint conditions. They are also helpful in the relief of stiff muscles, making them handy herbs for those of us who train too hard at any form of sport or exercise and regret it the following morning.

Topically, they make a wonderful ointment for drawing boils and abscesses, to remove toxins from the wounds, as well as to treat insect bites. They can be used as either an ointment or a poultice for this purpose.

**Folklore**    "Malva" is thought to come from the Greek word *malake*, meaning "soft", while the name "Althaea" derives from the Greek word *altho*, meaning "to cure". The ancient Greeks used the plant as a grave flower and planted it on the graves of loved ones, which is interesting in light of its association with Venus, and certainly a piece of lore that gives credence to my theory that it can also be associated with Inanna and related deities such as Freya. In the ancient world love was not so much the gentle thing it is often considered to be these days – love and death seem to have been far more closely connected.

The plant was known and esteemed by the ancient Greek physicians Dioscorides and Pliny.

According to Graves's *The White Goddess*, the flower was sacred to the goddess Althea, a garden fertility deity. According to the story, she hanged herself after hearing that her brothers had been killed by her son. Good old-fashioned family values certainly ran strong in the Greek myths!

A member of the mallow family was eaten as a vegetable by the Romans and the Egyptians.

The popular confectionery known as marshmallow used to be cooked from juice from the root of this herb – unfortunately that is no longer the practice with most commonly available marshmallows.

**Dose**    A tea made from 1 tsp of the herb infused into one cup of hot water can be taken three times a day. Take up to 4 ml of the tincture three times per day. A cold infusion of the root can be made by adding up to 4 g of the root to one cup of cold water – though this would certainly be a rather slimy cup to drink the following morning! The cold infusion does make a lovely wash for skin conditions, though, and can be drunk to soothe inflamed stomach conditions.

**Contraindications**    Taking too much can have a laxative effect. It is possible that the herb could delay the absorption of other drugs taken at the same time, due to its lining effect on the stomach, reducing space for medicines to absorb correctly, so leave at least two hours between taking conventional drugs and drinking marshmallow.

# Mallow recipes

## *Drawing ointment for boils, stings and splinters*

**Ingredients**
- » marshmallow leaves
- » plantain leaves (broad-leafed plantain works well)
- » organic seed or vegetable oil
- » beeswax

**Instructions**   Check the leaves and make sure they are completely dry, then shred them as finely as possible – a food processor may work well for this. Pack them into a double boiler and pour the seed oil over the top until the leaves have been covered. Please note that with this recipe it is impossible to give you an idea of how much fresh plant matter to use – it depends entirely on the size of the leaves, how much moisture they contain, and how bulky they are, which is why the suggestion is to finely chop them and then just cover them with the oil. Keep trickling oil over until it stops bubbling – that way you know that all the herbs have been covered. You can use dried herbs instead, but I don't find them to be quite as drawing in action. As with fresh herbs, just cover the dried herbs with the oil: you will find that you don't need as much oil for dried herbs as you do for fresh, as they take up less space.

Warm up the pan and allow to simmer gently for at least an hour, two if possible – keep an eye on it to make sure the lower pan doesn't boil dry. Filter off the resulting oil through muslin or kitchen towels and leave it in a heavy Pyrex jug for at least half a day, until the murky stuff has sunk to the bottom. Pour off the clear oil into a separate jug, and add 18 g of beeswax for every 100 ml (3½ fl oz) of oil. Warm the mixture back up in the double boiler, stirring until the beeswax has dissolved, then pour into jars.

To use, smear a really thick layer (at least 2 mm, if possible) on a large plaster with adhesive on all four sides – a clean, sterile dressing works well for this. Apply this poultice over any area that needs drawing – boils, abscesses, splinters and such like. Leave it for at least half a day, longer if possible, then check to see whether, say, the splinter has drawn free. Replace the poultice as often as needed. Keep the area warm to encourage boils to drain and splinters to come free.

## Marshmallow cold infusion

**Ingredients**
- » 1 large handful of fresh leaves and flowers, or a 2.5–5 cm (1–2 in.) piece of fresh root
- » 570 ml (20 fl oz) of water

**Instructions**    Wash the root thoroughly if you are using this, and finely chop or grate it before piling it into a Kilner jar. If you are using leaves and flowers, finely chop these using a mezzaluna, a pair of herb scissors or any other herb-chopping implement you prefer, and pile them into your jar. Pour over enough clean, fresh water to cover the herbs – 570 ml (20 fl oz) is usually a good amount. Put the lid on and put the jar into the fridge overnight. This method of preparing the herbs gently extracts the mucilage without damaging it – mucilage is often badly broken down by adding hot water to it.

## Marshmallow tincture

**Ingredients**
- » plenty of fresh, chopped or grated marshmallow root, or plenty of shredded fresh or dried mallow leaves and flowers
- » alcohol of your preference – vodka or brandy work well

**Instructions**    Marshmallow tinctures are very simple to make, and it is advisable to prepare two separate ones: one using the root, and one using the leaves and flowers. Simply finely chop or grate the clean root, pile it into a jar and pour over enough alcohol to cover it, with about an extra couple of centimetres of alcohol on top of the herbs. The same principle applies to the chopped leaves and flowers – make sure they are chopped finely, and pour over the alcohol. In this case, 40% proof or thereabouts should work well, as the extra water content will encourage the mucilage to extract into the alcohol. Let the whole lot steep for a fortnight or more, shaking it up every couple of days, then filter off the herbs and bottle the liquid that remains. Take 1 tsp (5 ml) of the tincture up to three times a day. Use the root for more digestive-related issues, and the leaves for lung complaints.

# Rose

## *Rosa*

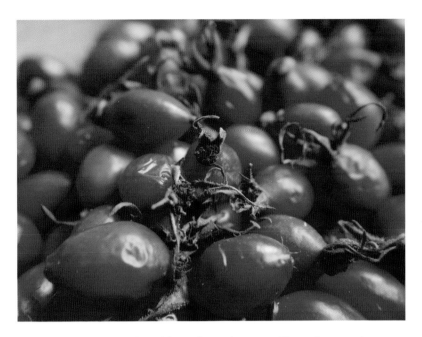

**Family**  Rosaceae, Rosoidae: damask rose (*Rosa damascena*);
apothecary's rose (*Rosa gallica*); ramanas rose (*Rosa rugosa*);
cabbage rose (*Rosa centifolia*); dog rose (*Rosa canina*); sweetbriar
(*Rosa rubiginosa*).

**Habitat and description**  Cultivated in gardens worldwide
for its well-known fragrance, the rose is thought to have
originated in Persia, although there are differing opinions on
this depending on the folklore and history examined. Roses
are still cultivated widely in Bulgaria for use in making attar
of roses. It is a popular garden plant in the UK, though the
hybrid tea roses mostly commonly seen in gardens are not
suitable for medicine. There are a variety of damask and Old
English roses, however, that provide highly scented petals that
can be used for medicine making.

Roses generally require good, fertile soil and plenty of sun to really produce the best blooms – my apothecary's rose currently sits in full sun and gives a good yield of flowers most years, especially when I speak gently to her whenever I pass and take care to give her plenty of plant food. Rose leaves are generally roughly ovoid and toothed, in opposite pairs up a slender stem with a single flower at the tip. The flowers range from five petals to dozens, depending on the species examined, and can span a wide range of colours, from white and palest pink to deep red, orange, yellow and even shades of purple. Roses generally have a generous endowment of thorns, so mind yourself while gathering them.

**Where to find it**    Apothecary's rose and related damask rose varieties can be grown in pretty much any temperate zone in the world, and in many countries that range more towards the hot side of the spectrum.

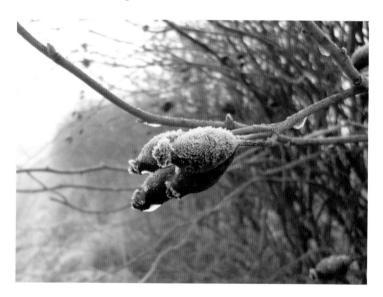

**Parts used**    Flowers, hips of damask and Old English roses.

**When to gather**    The petals when flowering; hips from September through February, depending on the type of rose.

**Medicines to make**    Sweets, jams and gummies; elixirs, wines, syrups, tinctures, teas, skin washes and infused oils; creams, salves and ointments.

**Constituents**    As with most herbs, roses contain a huge array of components, including (but not limited to): volatile oil containing beta-phenethyl alcohol, geraniol, nerol, citronellol, geranic acid, eugenol and myrcene.

**Planetary influence**    White roses are associated with the Moon, red with Jupiter.

**Associated deities and heroes**    Aphrodite, Venus, Freya and other deities linked with beauty and love.

**Festival**    Beltane and Midsummer.

**Constitution**    Cooling and drying.

**Actions and indications**    Rose is a gentle laxative and anti-inflammatory, and also has sedative, antidepressant, aphrodisiac and cardioactive actions. It can also be used as a mild local anaesthetic. It is used to treat high cholesterol levels, making it a lovely ingredient to combine with hawthorn flowers and berries – possibly not surprising, as they are members of the same plant family. Rose water – a by-product from the production of the essential oil – is a gentle skin astringent and makes an excellent toner for use in daily skincare, as well as a lovely addition to face creams and moisturisers and a gentle treatment for inflamed, tired eyes. Rose is also a cholagogue, is antiviral and is a menstrual regulator, possibly due to the combination of its gentle gallbladder-stimulant actions and its tonic action on the uterus.

   The herb can also be used to help depression and insomnia, calm anxiety and ease tension in the body and mind, and to relieve PMS. Rose petals can be used as a gentle decongestant for the womb, especially handy in relieving congestion and the associated pain and heavy menstrual flow. I also add it to recipes for fertility and to help a woman get in touch with her inner divine feminine, for which it is very useful. It is considered one of the specific herbs for uterine fibroids both for its affinity with the womb and for its astringent properties.

Rosehips, primarily of *Rosa canina,* are packed with vitamin C and anti-inflammatories, making them popular for musculoskeletal aches and pains, especially when combined with turmeric. They can be used to make a tasty syrup, elixir or honegar that can be taken on a daily basis as a prophylactic to ward off coughs and colds in preparation for winter. The vitamin C content can also help the body scavenge up free radicals and reduce the inflammation that causes and worsens so many diseases.

*Rosa rugosa* and *Rosa rubiginosa* are both also rather useful and fragrant.

**Folklore**    Apart from its well-known connections with beauty and love, the rose is also a symbol of secrecy and was once hung at meetings to indicate that no details spoken in confidence were to be revealed outside the room. This custom still continues in the ceiling roses found in older homes. There is a vast body of folklore surrounding the rose, dating from Greek and Roman times, such as the myth that red roses came about when Jupiter came across Venus bathing, the story being that the white roses growing nearby turned red in sympathy with her blushes. Another tale states that the roses became red when Cupid spilled red wine on them. Persian legends say that when the sun was born, the first rays that hit the ground created the first rose. This is only a very small amount of the lore associated with the rose – to cover it all would easily take up an entire book!

**Dose**   Rose jams and elixirs can be eaten or drunk in moderate doses of 10 ml per time, but do be aware that too much may have a laxative effect. Rose tincture can be taken in 5 ml doses up to four times a day.

**Contraindications**   Avoid using rose during pregnancy.

# Rose recipes

## *Rose and cider vinegar toner for acne-prone skin*

**Ingredients**
- » rose petals
- » cider vinegar
- » rose essential oil (if preferred)
- » rose water

**Instructions**   Pack a jar with fresh rose petals and pour over the unpasteurised cider vinegar. Pop the lid on and allow it to steep for at least two weeks, then strain out the petals and add an equal amount of rose water and 2–3 drops of rose essential oil, if you want to. This can be used as a toner as it is, or diluted down even more with extra rose water if you prefer. This sometimes stings the first time it is applied; however, it is very effective at reducing redness in the skin and lessening the likelihood of spots and acne. It can be used on all oily areas, such as across the face, the neck and upper chest, and the back and shoulders. For men, a version could be made using frankincense water instead of rose water and omitting the rose essential oil. You can use witch hazel instead of frankincense water if you prefer, but this can be very harsh and often too astringent on the skin, resulting in too much drying, prompting the body to produce too much oil again to over-compensate, which often makes the problem worse rather than better.

## *Rosehip syrup*

**Ingredients**

- » rosehips, as many as you want to gather – I use at least 2 pints, more if I have it
- » 3 lemons – juice and zest
- » 2.5 l (80 fl oz) of water
- » 3 star anise clusters, ground
- » 1 tsp (5 g) of cinnamon
- » 5 cm (2 in.) piece of fresh root ginger – or more if you prefer
- » 2 kg (4 lb 7 oz) of brown sugar

**Instructions**    If you can, gather the rosehips after a frost, so that the skins begin to break; if that isn't possible, pick them and pop them in the freezer overnight. This will make cooking them a good deal easier, so I strongly suggest not skipping this step if at all possible!

Put the rosehips into a large preserving pan and pour over 1.2 l (40 fl oz) of water, then add the zest and juice of the lemons (making sure the zest is well chopped first) plus the spices and the chopped ginger. Bring to a gentle simmer and allow to cook for an hour, mashing periodically. Turn off the heat and leave the rosehips overnight, then add another 1.2 l (40 fl oz) of water and bring the mixture back to a simmer for a further hour. Strain the whole lot through a double layer of muslin – this is important, as it will remove the little hairs that line the middle of the rosehip, which can be irritating to the stomach if ingested. Don't press the liquid through – instead, let it sit for a couple of hours to drip through slowly. Pour the resulting liquid back into the pan with the sugar and warm it gently until the sugar has dissolved, then bring it to a boil and boil it for 10 minutes, keeping a close eye on it. Once it has thickened slightly, take it off the heat and pour it into clean bottles. Put the lids on straight away – the heat from the syrup will encourage the bottles to "seal", which will help them to keep fresh for longer. Label the bottles when they are cool. Take 1 dessertspoonful (10 ml) of rosehip syrup once or twice a day, or use 1 tbsp (15 ml) in a mug of hot water to create a fragrant and tasty drink, perfect for chasing away the cold on chilly days. You can also pour this mixture over cakes and puddings, or use it in smoothies, porridge, overnight oats or a range of other recipes.

## Rosehip and turmeric joint ease

**Ingredients**
  » plenty of rosehips (approximately 2 pints works well)
  » fresh or dried turmeric root
  » black pepper
  » 2 lemons
  » brown sugar
  » 1.7 l (60 fl oz) of water (if making a syrup)
    *or*
  » vodka or brandy (if making an elixir)

**Instructions**   This remedy can be made as a syrup or an elixir. For both versions, first freeze the rosehips overnight, as you did with the rosehip syrup recipe. If you are making the syrup, put the rosehips into a heavy-based pan and add 1 tbsp, heaped, of dried turmeric root, or a large chunk of finely diced fresh turmeric root (5–8 cm works quite well). Add the zest and juice of 2 lemons and 1 tsp, heaped (up to 6 g), of ground black pepper, then pour over 1.2 l (40 fl oz) of water and bring to a gentle simmer. Be careful not to spill the resulting liquid on yourself or on any surfaces or tea towels, as turmeric has a habit of staining everything a delightful bright yellow! Simmer the mixture on low heat for at least an hour, stirring occasionally, then turn off the heat and leave it to steep overnight. The following day, add another 570 ml (20 fl oz) of water and simmer for 10 minutes, then strain the whole through a jelly bag. Add 500 g of sugar per 570 ml of the mixture and warm gently until the sugar has dissolved, then simmer for a few minutes, bottle and label. To start with, take 1 tsp (5 ml) of this mixture twice a day – be aware that in large doses turmeric can cause stomach ache, so starting with a low dose and working your way up is a good way to avoid unnecessary troubles! This blend is a tasty way to support good joint health through the winter. You can also add ground star anise or cinnamon, if you like.

To make the elixir, thaw the frozen rosehips, dice them finely, and put them, the turmeric root (chopped finely), the lemons and the black pepper into a Kilner jar. Pour over plenty of brandy – 700 ml (24½ fl oz) should work well. Add 200 g (7 oz) of brown sugar, and leave the whole lot to steep for a month. Filter the resulting elixir through a jelly bag to remove the fine hairs, and bottle. Take up to 1 tsp (5 ml) twice a day.

## Rosehip oxymel

**Ingredients**
- » plenty of fresh rosehips, harvested after the frost has softened them
- » unpasteurised cider vinegar, still with the mother in
- » local honey
- » spices according to preference: cinnamon, star anise and turmeric all work well, as does fresh root ginger

**Instructions**    Roughly chop up the rosehips and pile them into a Kilner jar, then pour over enough cider vinegar to cover the rosehips plus at least 4 centimetres on top. Add your choice of spices (finely ground) or finely grated ginger and turmeric (or all of the above, if you want to)! Don't forget to add plenty of local honey – I like to add at least 2 tbsp (30 ml or more) to this recipe, depending on how sweet you want the resulting oxymel. As the rosehips aren't cooked and broken down in this recipe, they retain their health-giving vitamin C content, which is good for boosting your immune system.

You can also do a version of this recipe as an alcohol-based elixir, using brandy, vodka or any other strong spirit – this has the benefit of being particularly warming. I tend to prefer a warming oxymel myself, because I run cold, though you may find that those who run warm will prefer the cooler vinegar-based versions.

## Rosehip and ginger honey

**Ingredients**
- » fresh rosehips after the frost has softened them
- » fresh root ginger
- » one large jar of local honey
- » plenty of patience!

**Instructions**    This is a bit of a fiddly recipe! First, chop off the very tip of each rosehip, removing the remains of the stamens. Then, using a sharp knife, slice the rosehips in half. Use a small spoon to scoop out and remove the seeds and irritating hairs from the middle of the rosehips, and chop them finely. Peel and finely grate the fresh root ginger – use as much as you want. Now thoroughly bash small batches of the rosehips and honey in a mortar and pestle, transferring each batch into a Kilner jar when you are happy that the ingredients are fully blended. Finally, stir in the grated root ginger. Leave the honey to steep for at least a fortnight.

You can pour dollops of this onto your breakfast porridge or granola, add it to smoothies, or just stir a spoonful into a cup of hot water. If you'd rather not have the bits of rosehip in, warm the honey gently (don't let it boil) and then pour it through a warm sieve, into a clean jar. It is important to pre-warm the sieve by pouring some boiling water through it first, as if you don't do this, the honey will thicken again on contact with the cold surface. The honey should drip through the warmed sieve, leaving the fruit and ginger behind, which can then be frozen in ice cube trays and added to chutney, jam or pickle recipes later on.

# Scots pine
## *Pinus sylvestris*

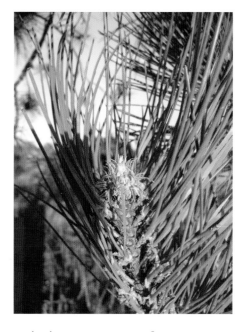

*Also known as:* Scots fir, Norway pine

**Family**   Pinaceae.

**Habitat and description**   A familiar sight in the UK, especially in Northern England and, of course, Scotland, as the
name suggests, Scots pine grows to a sturdy height of 45 m
(150 ft), with a trunk diameter of over 1.5 m (5 ft) in mature
specimens. Scots pine trees usually live for around 300 years,
though some trees reach double that age; there are exam-
ples in Finland that are over 700 years old. The needles are
evergreen, with fresh, bright-green young growth produced
in the spring at the ends of the twigs. Yellow or pink pollen
cones are produced in the spring, and the familiar pine cones

develop as the year progresses. These are shed from late autumn through the winter and make excellent kindling. The seeds are lightweight and papery and are formed between the scales of the pine cone – they are easily carried off by the wind and will settle wherever they can, forming young trees remarkably quickly. I have a pine growing in the guttering by my front door, where it has self-seeded from the mature trees at the bottom of the garden. Pine tends to prefer poorer soil, or boggy land – the ones in my garden grow right next to the stream, where they thrive. There are a number of subspecies in the Pine family, which developed in response to their particular area of growth – but in this instance we are examining the "parent" tree, *Pinus sylvestris*.

**Where to find it**   Native to Europe and the UK, Scots pine can be found ranging from Western Europe to Scandinavia; it copes with truly cold and snowy winters with aplomb.

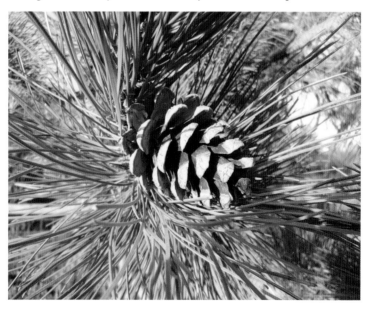

**Parts used**   Needles and pollen, resin; the bark is sometimes also used.

**When to gather**   All year round, as needed, for the needles; late spring and summer for the pollen.

**Medicines to make**   Decoctions and infusions; steams using the essential oil; infused vinegars and oils for salve making.

**Constituents**   Resins; volatile oils including alpha and beta pinene, limonene, chamazulene and others.

**Planetary influence**   Mars.

**Associated deities and heroes**   Cybele, Cernunnos, Pan, Herne and assorted Sun Gods, plus deities linked with the Winter Solstice.

**Festival**   Yule / Winter Solstice.

**Constitution**   Hot and dry.

**Actions and indications**   Scots pine is best known for its antiseptic and decongestant properties when used internally, rendering it very useful in the treatment of a variety of chest and upper-respiratory-tract ailments, including tuberculosis and pneumonia, bronchitis, colds, influenza and others. It acts as an expectorant when used as a steam, helping the body to remove excess phlegm and reduce the amount of phlegm produced. If you want to use Scots pine as a steam, add 1–2 drops of the essential oil to a bowl of hot water and lean over it with a towel covering your head and the bowl. Keep your eyes closed and inhale carefully through the nose to pull the evaporating essential oil down into your chest. Repeat this process twice a day to relieve sinusitis and chest complaints, particularly those with a hoarse cough and tight chest due to excess phlegm production.

Topically, Scots pine can be used as a balm or rub to reduce muscle stiffness and rheumatism, as well as to relieve neuralgia and sciatica, by pulling blood to the area. Make a Scots-pine infused oil, adding a few drops of extra pine essential oil once infusion has finished, and apply it twice a day, rubbing the area thoroughly to amplify the effects.

Pine needles are rich in vitamin C and have been used to treat cases of scurvy. These days they are used for their anti-oxidant properties; they make a very tasty salad dressing when infused in vinegar.

Pine-needle decoctions poured into the bath or rubbed onto the skin can be useful for the relief of a range of skin disorders, including itching or pruritis, eczema and psoriasis. These decoctions have also been used in the past to relieve bladder and kidney problems.

**Folklore**    The slain God Attis turned himself into a pine tree after his death. Pine trees were decorated and brought into temples dedicated to Cybele at the Spring Equinox, and seeds from the pine were used to brew ritual drinks. The tree is also linked with Dionysus, who carried a pine wand.

Pine is traditionally linked with death and immortality and has been an important part of funeral rites around the world. Some religions will only bury the dead in caskets made of pine wood. The tree is also associated with rebirth. The Celts linked it with the Warrior's Path, and it is one of the Ogham runes. The cones have been used in folk magic to boost women's fertility, and the tree was linked with Demeter for this purpose.

Resin from pine is used to create turpentine, which is a valuable and useful substance used to caulk ships, create varnishes, clean brushes in oil painting and for a host of other uses. Rosin is another by-product from the creation of turpentine – it is used on violin and cello bows. Pine is also used to create pitch and tar – the latter is gained from the tree roots, so the process is destructive.

**Dose**    Topically, use it as needed. To use internally, I recommend making a decoction: 1 tbsp of pine needles chopped and boiled in 570 ml (20 fl oz) of water – take doses of 1 tbsp

(15 ml) up to three times a day. Tinctures are not easy for the home-medicine maker to achieve, as the resins will only extract in very strong alcohol – ideally 90% proof.

**Contraindications**   Can cause contact dermatitis in some people.

# Scots pine recipes

## Scots-pine infused vinegar

**Ingredients**
» at least 2 handfuls of fresh Scots pine needles
» balsamic vinegar

**Instructions**   Finely chop the Scots pine needles and pack them into a Kilner jar, then pour over the balsamic vinegar until it just covers the leaves. Pop the top on and leave it to steep for at least a month – I left mine for a good six months, and it really made for a great flavour. Strain out the needles after this time and bottle the vinegar, letting it sit for another six months to mature. This vinegar can be added to salad dressings, houmous and any other recipes you like a good savoury vinegar in, and it has the added benefit that the vitamin C content of the pine needles has not been broken down by heat.

## Scots pine syrup

**Ingredients**
» 1 pint of loosely packed Scots pine needles – I have used them all year round, though the very young, bright-green growth produced in spring has a delicious flavour
» 1.2 l (40 fl oz) of water

- »  1 unwaxed lemon
- »  1 lime
- »  500 g (1 lb 1½ oz) sugar – preferably organic or Fairtrade

**Instructions**   Roughly chop the Scots pine needles and put them into a saucepan with the zest and juice of the lemon and lime, then bring the whole lot to a simmer, keeping a lid on the pan. Let it simmer for at least 30 minutes – it may take longer than this as the needles are resinous and will not give up their goodness easily. Once the liquid smells piney as well as citrusy, strain out the herbs and fruit, then pour the liquid back into the pan and add the sugar. Simmer gently and stir the mixture until the sugar has melted, then boil quickly for 5 minutes before bottling. Enjoy a spoonful daily to boost vitamin C levels and as an expectorant when you have colds or flu.

## Scots-pine infused oil

**Ingredients**
- »  1 pint of loosely packed Scots pine needles, gathered as needed
- »  organic oil: rapeseed, olive, sunflower or sweet almond all work well

**Instructions**   This recipe can be made either in a double boiler – which can be perched on top of a wood-burning stove at this time of the year – or in a slow cooker. The resin content in the needles needs long, slow infusion to extract fully into the oil, so expect this recipe to take a while! Use a mezzaluna to finely chop the needles and, if you are using a slow cooker, pile them in and pour over enough oil to cover the needles. Put the lid on and let it simmer on low for at least six hours, preferably longer – this oil is often best left for a full day, or overnight. Alternatively, you can infuse your oil with the finely chopped needles in a double boiler on a wood-burning stove, but this will need to be left simmering gently for several hours. Keep an eye on the water level, as if the lower pan boils dry, it can damage the pan.

Once the oil has infused and you can smell the pine in it, strain out the herbs through a piece of kitchen roll and add a couple of extra drops of pine essential oil. Bottle the infused oil and label it carefully. This can be used as a massage oil for sore muscles after heavy sports or exercise or for rheumatism and arthritis, or rubbed onto the chest and back for chest infections. You can also turn this oil into a plaister by adding 18 g of beeswax per 100 ml (3½ fl oz) of oil, melting the whole lot down and pouring it onto squares of fabric which, once set, can be bandaged to the joint in question.

# Silverweed
## *Potentilla anserina*

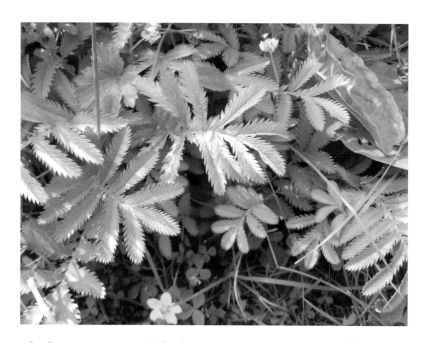

*Also known as:* prince's feathers, goosewort, silvery cinquefoil, moor grass, wild agrimony, trailing tansy, wild tansy, goose grey, argentia, five leaf grass, crampweed

**Family**  Rosaceae.

**Habitat and description**  This stunning little plant was one of my first encounters when I began to look seriously at the wildflowers around me and to try to identify them. I was at school in Kent at the time, and my class and I were taken on a day trip to the Seven Sisters, in Sussex, to work on some geography exercises. While I was there, I found an enchanting little silvery-leafed beauty growing plentifully in the grass, and, spending far more time examining the plant than actually working on my exercises, I ended up picking several leaves to take home with me.

Silverweed likes to grow in grass, I have found, and especially in places that flood regularly over the winter, making it an interesting marker for those places that get particularly soggy underfoot when the weather turns. It can also be found growing on chalky or sandy soils. A close relative of tormentil and agrimony, as well as cinquefoil, the plant has beautiful silvery-toothed leaves in opposite pairs on stems up to 12.5 cm (5 in) long, and the leaves are covered in soft velvet on both sides. The flowers, found from May through to September, look rather like those of a buttercup, but they are a gentler yellow and are covered in the same velvet as the leaves. The yellow against all the silver is a lovely sight! If you grow silverweed in your garden, don't be too surprised if it wanders outside the herb garden by way of the long underground runners it sends out to propagate itself. During rainy weather the leaves crowd together and protect the yellow flowers, which also close. The root used to be used as a famine food, and if you dig up a silverweed plant, you will find a surprisingly substantial-looking root that can be dried and ground as a flour substitute. It is still used for this purpose in Tibet.

**Where to find it**   Most temperate regions of the world, including the UK and Europe, and countries further afield, such as Tibet.

**Parts used**   The leaves and roots. Previously, the seeds were also used.

**When to gather**   Midsummer for the leaves, autumn for the roots.

**Medicines to make**    Infused oils, balms, tinctures, milk infusions, standard infusions and decoctions; flour from the roots; powder.

**Constituents**    Ellagitannins, including catechins; flavonoids, including astragalin and quercetin; coumarins; umbelliferone and scopoletin.

**Planetary influence**    Moon.

**Associated deities and heroes**    Virgin Mary, and most of the Moon and Mother Goddesses.

**Festival**    Not known, though potentially Midsummer, as this is when the plant is usually in flower.

**Constitution**    Cool and dry.

**Actions and indications**    Perhaps one of the main uses for silverweed is as a superb astringent, due to its high tannin content – up to 25% by weight. This makes it useful for any

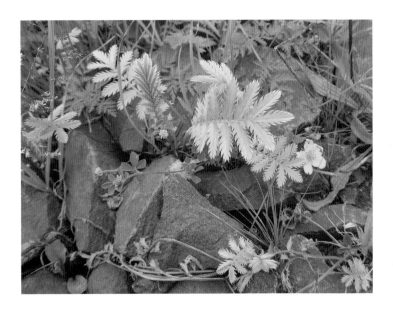

lax conditions of the mucous membranes, from diarrhoea to bleeding and haemorrhage. Topically, silverweed can also be used to stop piles bleeding and encourage them to shrink, and as a gargle for sore throats.

Traditionally, this herb has been used as a wound poultice, particularly for wounds that are stubborn to heal. The herb was boiled in milk, and the milk drunk to prevent sepsis, while the mashed herbs were applied to the wound as a poultice.

Silverweed has an affinity with the bladder and kidneys and can be helpful in the relief of urinary gravel, its antispasmodic properties providing relief to the discomfort associated with this condition. As an extension of this, it can be used to relieve griping, spasmodic pains of the stomach, the digestive tract as a whole, and also the uterus. It can prove very helpful in relieving painful and heavy periods, especially as the menopause approaches.

Silverweed has been used in the past to make a mouthwash for mouth ulcers, bleeding and spongy gums and loose teeth, and can also be used to save the gums and teeth in cases of scurvy, where the astringent and wound-healing properties of this herb come in very handy.

The high tannin content of silverweed has been shown to have anti-mutagenic properties.

**Folklore**   Silverweed was previously used as a fomentation for smallpox, to stop scarring. A piece of German folklore holds that this plant is a favourite of the Good Neighbours, and that the Faery folk will spend their nights chatting and laughing while seated on the leaves of silverweed. Who can blame them, considering how soft and beautiful the leaves are!

**Dose**   I recommend 2–4 ml of the tincture up to three times a day. Alternatively, use 1 tsp of chopped herb to a cup of hot water, up to three times a day.

**Contraindications**   None known at present.

# Silverweed recipes

## Silverweed and toadflax pile balm

**Ingredients**
- » ½ pint each of silverweed and toadflax, gathered in late summer or early autumn, or 25 g each of the dried herbs
- » organic seed oil
- » beeswax

**Instructions**    As with most of the ointment and balm recipes, make sure the herbs are clean and dry, then chop them finely and pile them into the top of a double boiler, covering them with just enough oil to cover the herbs. Infuse it on a moderate heat for an hour, then strain out the herbs and repeat the process with a fresh batch of herbs for a really strong, astringent balm. Filter out the second lot of herbs and add 12 g of beeswax to each 100 ml (3½ fl oz) of oil. Return the lot to the heat and stir it until the wax has melted, then pour the concoction into little jars. Label them and put the lids on. This balm can be used for piles, and it has been left unfragranced for this purpose, as it will be used on or near a very sensitive area – better safe than sorry (or sore!). The balm can also be used for varicose veins, and for this use it can have a fragrance added, if preferred.

## Silverweed poultice for wounds

**Ingredients**
- » 1 large handful of fresh silverweed
- » 1 tbsp (15 ml) of boiling water

**Instructions**    Shred the leaves, if possible, and pile them into a food processor, adding the hot water and blitzing until you have a thick pulp. Scoop this out and smear it onto a clean piece of cloth, applying it to the wound in question and leaving it in place for half an hour to dry it out and encourage it to heal cleanly.

If you don't have a food processor, you can either chew the leaves and make a spit poultice out of them, which can then be applied to the cut or graze in question, or you can finely chop the leaves and then bash them thoroughly using a mortar and pestle, after which the process is the same as described above.

Silverweed poultice can be used for stubborn cuts or grazes that just won't close, in order to draw the edges together and encourage healing.

## Silverweed tincture

**Ingredients**
- » plenty of fresh silverweed leaves
- » brandy or vodka

**Instructions**    As with most of the tincture recipes mentioned already, simply finely chop the leaves and flowers, pile them into a clean Kilner jar, and pour over enough alcohol to cover the herbs with 1 cm of liquid over the top of the leaves. Let the whole thing infuse for at least a fortnight, then strain out the herbs. Take 1 tsp (5 ml) of this tincture once or twice a day for any wet, inflamed conditions, including diarrhoea, for excessive menstruation, and also as a general-purpose kidney and bladder tonic.

## Silverweed flour

**Ingredients**
- » plenty of fresh silverweed roots

**Instructions**    Scrub the roots clean and roughly dry them using a clean cloth, then slice them fairly thinly and dry the slices in a dehydrator. Using a mortar and pestle or a coffee grinder, grind the dried root slices into as fine a powder as possible, after which you can add it to recipes requiring flour – either as is, or mixed with other flour, if you want. It can be stored in an airtight jar in a cool, dry place.

# Solomon's seal
## *Polygonatum multiflorum*

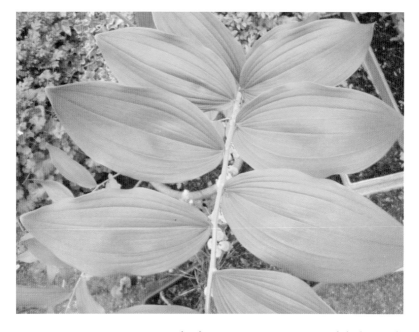

*Also known as:*  St Mary's seal, lady's seals

**Family**  Liliaceae.

**Habitat and description**  Solomon's seal is a woodland native of North America and Europe; it is commonly cultivated as a garden plant here in the UK, where it thrives in partial shade and good, moist soils. It grows from a central corm that produces the main medicinal rhizome, forming long, knotted growths underground reaching out horizontally. Each stem leaves behind a scar on the rhizome, which, when dug up, is quite similar to the colour of old bone and is juicy and fairly easy to cut up. The plant seems to produce one extra stem for each year of life – the one in my garden at present is eight years old, and will most likely produce eight or nine stems next spring if it continues to follow patterns established to date. These new stems only start to appear fairly late on in spring, making it easy to assume the plant has died over the winter – but just as you have given up hope of the plant re-emerging, you will find that solid green shoots begin to poke through the soil. These rapidly grow to form graceful arches, with roughly ovate, veined leaves growing alternately up the stem, beginning about two thirds of the way up. These give rise to clusters of beautiful, waxy flowers in late spring and early summer that are bone white, yellow white and palest green in colour, hanging in downward-facing bells from the stem. These then produce blue-black berries, each containing several seeds. The flowers are delightfully fragrant, but you do need to get down on your knees by the plant to fully appreciate the scent, a practice that I wholeheartedly recommend.

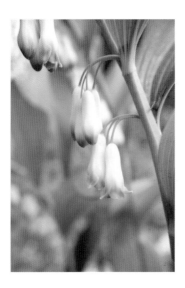

**Where to find it**    North America, Asia, Northern Europe and parts of the UK, where it has naturalised. Garden escapees can also be found quite commonly.

**Parts used**    The root, rhizome and side roots are the parts most often used. The berries are, however, poisonous so should not be used.

**When to gather**    Autumn and winter, once the plant has gone dormant. Only take part of the root – allow the plant plenty of root to regrow from.

**Medicines to make**    Tinctures and elixirs, root powders and decoctions.

**Constituents**    Saponins and lectins; convallarin, asparagine, sugar, pectin and starch – tinctures made from the plant often end up quite thick and syrupy; mucilage and saponins.

**Planetary influence**    Saturn.

**Associated deities and heroes**    Commonly linked with King Solomon, and also the Virgin Mary – by extension, I suspect it could also be linked with many Moon Goddesses.

**Festival**    None known at present.

**Constitution**    Cold and moist.

**Actions and indications**    Solomon's seal has not seen a huge amount of use over here in the UK, but it has a long tradition of use in North America. The plant is another of those fantastic herbs that manages to blend astringent, demulcent and tonic properties, making it healing and restorative to a variety of areas of the body and the issues that affect them.

It is best known for its effects on bones and joints – the root decoction has long been taken to help bones knit cleanly and correctly, both when used internally and when applied externally. The plant is also great for tendons and ligaments, as it teaches proper elasticity, helping connective tissue to function at optimum; this makes it very useful for repeat injuries or injuries where tendons and ligaments have become over-stretched and have not healed back to correct length and flexibility. The root, used internally and externally, both moistens and soothes, restoring tone. It has also been used to remove bone spurs and bunions, especially those caused by excess and damaging pressure on joints – by regulating tendon and ligament length and function, it removes the excess pressure that is causing the problem, and then helps the body to remove the bone spurs themselves. In addition, it can be used to relieve issues of internal prolapse due to tendon laxness, such as uterine prolapse after birth. For more in-depth information on this plant, I highly recommend Matthew Wood's excellent books (see Recommended Reading).

The root isn't just used for the tendons and bones, however – it can also be used to relieve bleeding of the lungs and inflammatory conditions of the stomach and bowels, where its mucilage and vulnerary content encourage healing and relieve pain. It is a tonic to digestion and has been used to heal fatty liver and act as a liver protective.

The root has a regulating effect on heart muscle due to the presence of convallarin, found in trace amounts. (Much higher quantities are found in its relative, lily of the valley, but this should only be used with medical advice.) Regulating the heart muscle can also have a positive effect on the mind, calming anxiety and stress where this is due to the heart and digestion functioning poorly.

Topically, the powdered roots have long been used for bruises, piles and inflammation. The leaves and roots can be made into a cream for black eyes and bruising and also to act as both a drawing poultice and a wound healer, due to the presence of mucilage and tannins. If you want to make an ointment, you'll need to thinly slice and dry the root before powdering it.

Distilled water made from the flowers has previously been used in Italy for purifying the skin and removing freckles and marks – it would make an excellent addition to a cream, if made using an alembic.

**Folklore**    The roots contain a lot of pectin and mucilage, and have in the past been boiled in water to produce a food substance. The young shoots have been boiled and eaten as a vegetable, and the root can be powdered and used as a bread substitute in times of famine.

Solomon's seal is one of the roots referred to as "High John the Conqueror" – referring to High John, an escaped slave in the Deep South who managed to avoid recapture through the use of conjuring and magic, and was afterwards much known for using conjuring to aid those poor folk still enslaved on the plantation.

**Dose**    Drop doses of 10 drops of tincture twice a day works well. Alternatively, I also use a dose of 1 tbsp (15 ml) in a week's worth of medicine to good effect.

**Contraindications**    The berries are highly toxic and should not be used. The leaves can cause nausea if chewed – they are generally used for topical preparations only.

# Solomon's seal recipes

## Solomon's seal cream

**Ingredients**

- » 3–4 in. (7.5–10 cm) of fresh root, or 2 tbsp of dried, powdered root
- » Solomon's seal aromatic flower water (optional)
- » organic seed oil
- » beeswax
- » organic vegetable glycerine
- » vitamin E oil
- » chamomile essential oil

**Instructions**    If you are using fresh root, you need to clean it thoroughly after unearthing it, using a small toothbrush or nailbrush to get into all the nooks and crannies. Dry the root as thoroughly as you can, then slice it as thinly as possible, before putting the slices into a dehydrator on a low setting or into a very low oven, until the surface is fairly dry – check back every 10 minutes to avoid drying the roots out completely. The idea here is to remove the surface water without damaging the mucilage content too much, so you don't want the root to be dry all the way through. Once the root is surface dry, slice it into thin matchsticks and pile it into the top of a double boiler or into a slow cooker. If, rather than starting with fresh root, you are using dried, powdered root to make the cream, just put 2 tablespoons of dried root into the double-boiler top or the slow cooker.

Cover the root with at least 250 ml (9 fl oz) organic vegetable seed oil and heat over a pan of simmering water in the double boiler for at least an hour. This stage can also be done in a slow cooker, where it can be left for a full day to infuse – this works well as you get a stronger oil if you can infuse it for much longer, and slow cookers can be left without the need for constant checking. Long infusion will draw out more of the root's properties; roots are quite a bit more tough than leaves so they often take at least double the infusion time to get a good, effective infused oil.

Once you are happy with the strength of the oil, strain it through muslin or kitchen roll, then set it to one side. Measure out 200 ml (7 fl oz) of the oil, and add 15 g of beeswax, returning both ingredients to the double boiler. If you used a slow cooker to make the oil, you will need to move it into a double boiler at this point, as a double boiler heats much faster than a slow cooker.

Before you turn it back on to heat, however, prepare a root decoction: add 1 tbsp of dried or 2 tbsp of finely chopped fresh root to 570 ml (20 fl oz) of filtered water in a clean saucepan. Cover and simmer gently for 10 minutes. You could do a cold infusion instead, but remember that mucilage is destroyed by heat – you will still need to heat your cold infusion in order to get it to properly emulsify with the oil, as both liquids need to be approximately the same temperature in order to mix properly, and so I recommend simply making a standard hot decoction of the root. Alternatively, if you have a flower water made using the flowers from the plant, you can use that instead of a root decoction or cold infusion. Once you are happy with the decoction of the root, strain it through coffee-filter paper, measure out 200 ml (7 fl oz) of it and put it back into the clean pan, adding 2 tsp (10 ml) of organic vegetable glycerine. Put this aside for the moment.

Now return the oil and beeswax mix in the double boiler to the heat and warm it through until the wax has melted, then pour it into a clean, dry food processor. Put the pan with the decoction or the flower water and glycerine mixture in it back on to a gentle heat if it has cooled too much, stirring until the glycerine has fully dissolved and has mixed well with the decoction or mixture. Keep an eye on the oil and wax mix in the food processor – once it has cooled enough to turn opaque but still moves freely when you move the processor dish, you are ready to begin blending the cream. Turn the motor onto a low or moderate setting, then pour a steady, small trickle of the glycerine water into the oil mixture. Pause the process every minute or so to scrape down the sides and make sure that the mixture is emulsifying properly. Keep mixing until the glycerine water has blended thoroughly with the oil mixture. Once you are happy with it, add 5 drops of vitamin E oil and 5 drops of chamomile essential oil per 100 ml (3½ fl oz) of cream, and give it another quick blend to mix it in thoroughly. Scrape the mixture into clean, sterile jars fairly quickly – it will thicken as it sets, which makes it much harder to pour neatly. Store this cream in the fridge and use it for any bruises, bumps, strains, sprains, or damaged or pulled ligaments and tendons, and even for bunions, bone spurs and other joint- or bone-related issues. It will keep for up to six weeks, though I have known creams to keep for much longer than that – smell it regularly, and as long as it looks and smells ok, it should be absolutely fine to use. Don't forget to label it – I do recommend putting a couple of suggestions for usage on the jar if possible, as well as the date of making it.

## Solomon's seal drawing poultice

**Ingredients**
- » fresh Solomon's seal root
- » local honey – preferably set

**Instructions**    This is a bit of an odd recipe, combining the properties of set honey and fresh Solomon's seal root. Dig up the root and scrub it thoroughly, then dry the surface as much as you can before finely dicing the root or, if possible, grating it on the finest setting you have. Pile the root gratings into a bowl and add a small dollop of set honey, then use a fork to work the root shavings into the honey until they are evenly mixed. Ideally you want to aim for at least half of the mix being root, and half honey. The honey has preserving properties as well as adding its own drawing effects to the poultice. Pack the poultice into a clean jar, label it carefully, and store in the fridge; alternatively, if you don't think you will use it fairly quickly, freeze it in ice-cube trays. Ideally, this poultice needs to be used within two weeks if stored in the fridge, because the honey content isn't high enough to preserve it for longer. You can also prepare this recipe with runny honey, which is better if you plan to use the honey internally – but set honey melts more slowly in contact with the skin, making the drawing properties of the poultice a bit longer lasting. If you want to prepare your poultice using only a small amount of honey – just enough to stick the root shavings together – and you are worried that it will not keep, try packing it into ice-cube trays in the freezer. Once fully frozen, pop them into a labelled tub or resealable food bag; they can then be defrosted as needed. To use the poultice, smear it onto a generous square of thick muslin and apply it to any area that needs grit or muck pulling out of wounds. I suspect you could also poultice breaks, strains and sprains with this mixture to encourage the bones, joints or ligaments to heal cleanly.

Alternatively, try making a standard ointment with the grated root: following a similar procedure to the first part of the cream recipe above, simply grate or chop the fresh, surface-dry root and give it a long, slow infuse into oil. Strain the mixture, then add 18 g of beeswax per 100 ml (3½ fl oz) of oil this time, to make a much thicker set. Stir this in a double boiler until melted, then pour into jars. This can be smeared onto plasters and applied to mucky cuts or grazes. The advantage of the honey recipe, however, is that by not heating the root, the mucilage is left intact, making it a bit more effective as a drawing poultice.

## Solomon's seal tincture

**Ingredients**
» Solomon's seal root – as much as you have available, although remember to leave plenty for the plant to regrow from
» brandy, vodka or gin, as strong as you can get

**Instructions**   This was one of the first root tinctures I attempted, many years ago, and I have fond memories of it even now! Solomon's seal roots are surprisingly reminiscent of bones – vertebrae, or even finger joints and bones – giving an interesting sign of the things it can help us with. Once you have unearthed the roots, scrub them thoroughly, then finely chop or grate them before packing them into a Kilner jar. Pour over the alcohol, adding an extra few centimetres on top of the root. Leave the mixture to steep for at least a fortnight. When you check it again, you will almost certainly find that the liquid has gone thick and almost syrupy – this is the mucilage content extracting into the water. If you don't want this, you will need to use stronger alcohol, but the mucilage content is so useful in itself that I suspect you'll be happy to see it. The resulting tincture, when strained, is sweet, nourishing, rooty and earthy, with a slightly bitter aftertaste, and it can be taken in drops or up to 20 ml added to a week's worth of medicine.

# Sweet cicely
## *Myrrhis odorata*

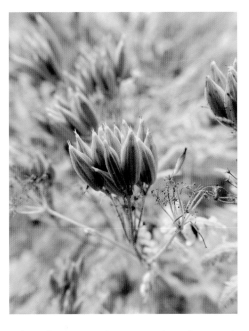

*Also known as:* greater chervil, Roman plant, cow chervil, smooth cicely, sweet fern, British myrrh, shepherd's needle, sweets, fern-leaved chervil, wild myrrh, sweet cus, sweet hemlock, beaked parsley

**Family** Apiaceae.

**Habitat and description** Sweet cicely is an attractive plant that grows in herb gardens and hedgerows across Britain. It has feathery leaves, much like those of cow parsley, with similar umbels of white flowers in the summer. The whole plant is strongly aromatic, with a large, thick root and a plethora of rather attractive filmy foliage in May. It is a hardy, herbaceous perennial that can grow up to 1 m (3 ft) tall. The plant prefers a soil rich in humus, and likes light shade. I have grown it very easily in tubs as well.

This is a robust little plant, and its flowers are followed by large dark seeds that make it stand out from the other members of the Apiaceae family, which includes many downright dangerous plants. An alternative name for the family is Umbelliferae, derived from the parasol shape of the flower clusters. The plant can often be found growing in grassy places, hedgerows, woodlands and hilly areas. It has a large, thick, hollow tap root and feathery leaves, which turn a shade of purple during the autumn. The ripe seeds slightly resemble those of plants such as fennel and dill, being dark brown, glossy and ridged in appearance, although they are somewhat larger in size than the aforementioned herb seeds.

Because this plant so closely resembles a number of thoroughly unpleasant poisonous plants, I strongly advise that you do not forage sweet cicely from the hedgerows. Buy a plant for your garden instead!

**Where to find it**    Native to Central and Southern Europe, and commonly found wild in the UK from parts of Yorkshire up to Scotland.

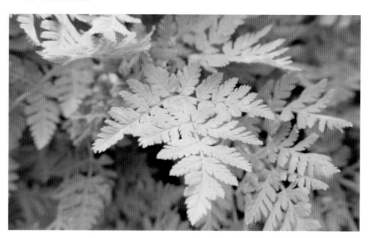

**Parts used**    Seeds, leaves and root.

**When to gather**    Autumn, and summer.

**Medicines to make**    Teas, tinctures, infused wines; a form of sweetener made from the dried leaves; infused oils, balms and poultices.

**Constituents**    Sweet cicely contains a range of constituents, some of which are reputedly similar to those from liquorice (*Glycyrrhiza glabra*), possibly giving rise to its reputation as an adaptogen. The plant contains a volatile oil that is composed of a range of constituents, including limonene. It also contains flavonoids such as luteolin and apigenin glucosides.

**Planetary influence**    Jupiter.

**Associated deities and heroes**    The plant is sacred to the Virgin Mary, St Cecilia and the Summer Goddess, as well as other deities associated with plants and fertility. As the plant acts in such a benign, warming way, some of the more benign Sun Gods and Goddesses could be linked.

**Festival**    Midsummer.

**Constitution**    Warm and dry.

**Actions and indications**    Sweet cicely is a gentle stomachic and tonic. The dried root can be used as a decoction for coughs and flatulence, and the herb can be infused to treat anaemia and act as a general tonic. It was used alongside angelica as a prophylactic during the Great Plague.

It has also been used in the past to treat hypertension, and the leaves were used as a diuretic. It is not used a great deal these days, which is rather a shame for such a gentle and tasty plant.

The whole plant has been used as an anti-infective, and a decoction of the root can be used to treat tuberculosis. It is a gentle emmenagogue and galactagogue, as well as a nervine tonic. The whole herb can be used to treat stomach weakness, especially where this is due to coldness or the presence of too much phlegm, as it is gently warming, drying and stimulating. The diuretic properties make it useful for the treatment of gout, for which it was much used in the past.

Earlier in historical use, Culpeper stated that "the root boiled, and eaten with oil and vinegar . . . do much warm and please old and cold stomachs." He also stated that the plant can be used to bring on the menses and encourage the passing of afterbirth, as well as to treat diseases of the lungs. He reckons that the whole plant is so mild that anyone can use it. John Gerard agreed with Culpeper, stating that it could be used "for old people that are dull and without courage: it rejoiceth and comforteth the heart, and increases their lust and strength". It certainly is a warming, heartening plant!

The root is antibacterial, perhaps where its reputation as an anti-plague herb came from.

It has been used as a gentle stimulant for debilitated stomachs, and is a valuable tonic for 15- to 18-year-old girls – particularly those of a more melancholy or weepy disposition. The distilled water has been used as a diuretic and is helpful in pleurisy. The essence of the plant is aphrodisiac, and a decoction of the root in wine, when taken in the morning and evening, is apparently effective for the treatment of consumption.

Externally, the plant can be used as an ointment to treat green wounds and open and foul-smelling ulcers and to ease the pain of gout. The plant contains either glycyrrhizin or a very similar substance, which could account partly for the herb's reputation as an adaptogen.

It is a wonderful tonic for those facing exhaustion, and to help recuperation after a long illness, as it gently warms and strengthens the whole system and helps the body to regain and maintain equilibrium. All in all, sweet cicely is a fantastic and much-loved herb, useful and gentle, and one that has been rather forgotten in recent years, though perhaps it is time for it to make a comeback!

**Folklore**    There isn't a great deal of folklore surrounding this herb that is part of common knowledge. However, it is known that the Latin name for the plant comes from the Greek *myrrhis*, meaning "smelling of myrrh", with the specific name "odorata" deriving from the Latin word *odorus*, meaning "fragrant". Several of the common names of the plant reflect this.

**Dose**    1 tsp of dried herb to a cup of hot water, taken three times a day.

**Contraindications**    None have been found; however, it would be sensible to use this herb with great caution during pregnancy, due to its emmenagogue properties.

# Sweet cicely recipes

## Sweet cicely infused wine

### Ingredients
- » 1 handful of sweet cicely leaves
- » ½ handful of green sweet cicely seeds
- » 1 piece of sweet cicely root (optional)
- » 1 bottle of red or white wine, as you prefer
- » maple syrup

**Instructions**    Check over the leaves and dice them roughly, and then pulverise the seeds using a mortar and pestle until they are well broken down. Pile the ingredients into a large jar, add a spoonful of maple syrup if you want a sweet tonic wine, then pour in the bottle of wine. Leave it to steep for a few days, then have approximately 150 ml (5 fl oz) every evening for a few days to act as a gentle digestive tonic.

## Sweet cicely honey

### Ingredients

- » 1 large handful of fresh sweet cicely leaves
- » one jar of local runny honey
- » ½ handful of green sweet cicely seeds (optional)

**Instructions**    Finely dice the leaves as small as you can and stir them into a jar of local runny honey – you may need to decant the whole thing into a larger jar to fit it all in. If you have the green seeds, you can finely chop these and add them. Green sweet cicely seeds are better for use than brown seeds, as once the seeds turn brown, they have lost most of their aroma and flavour – better to keep these to sow for more plants next year. Let the honey infuse for at least a week. Both the leaves and the chopped green seeds can be eaten as they are, direct from the jar, or you can grind them up further using a mortar and pestle, honey and all, before using them in other recipes. Take 1 tsp (5 ml) doses of the honey as a digestive tonic, or use it to sweeten teas and liven up cakes, puddings and desserts.

## Sweet cicely plaister

### Ingredients / equipment

- » 2 large handfuls of the fresh sweet cicely leaves
- » organic seed oil
- » beeswax
- » 10 in. (25 cm) squares of cloth – old towel or tea towel works well

**Instructions**    Finely chop the sweet cicely leaves and infuse them in the oil using a double boiler for at least an hour, then strain out the herbs and add 16 g of beeswax per 100 ml

(3½ fl oz) of oil. Heat again until the wax has melted, then stir to mix it thoroughly with the oil. Pour the resulting liquid onto the squares of cloth laid onto plates, leave them to cool, then lift the ointment-soaked fabric off the plates and lay them onto large rectangles of greaseproof paper, allowing at least 5 cm (2 in.) of extra paper on two opposite sides of the fabric, and a width of extra paper equal to the width of the fabric on the other two sides, so that you can fold it over and completely cover the plaister. Scrape off the remainder of the ointment stuck to the plate and smear it onto the plaister, then fold the two larger ends of greaseproof paper over the fabric, and roll the whole thing up loosely. Store them in jam jars, or use a rubber band to hold the greaseproof paper together. Keep them out of the heat, and don't forget to label them carefully. The plaisters can be applied to rheumatic or arthritic joints and can also be used in cases of gout.

## Sweet cicely and self heal recuperative tonic

**Ingredients**
- » fresh sweet cicely root
- » dried or fresh self heal flowering tops
- » brandy
- » honey or maple syrup

**Instructions**  Finely chop the sweet cicely root and put it into a Kilner jar, then shred and pour in an equivalent amount of dried self heal flowering tops, pour over enough brandy to cover the herbs, and add 1 large tablespoonful of honey or maple syrup. Shake the mixture up and leave it to steep for a fortnight, then strain out the herbs and bottle the resulting mixture. If you want to use fresh self heal rather than dried, prepare the concoction with just the sweet cicely root and leave it in the jar until the self heal is flowering, then add plenty of finely chopped flowering tops and steep for another two weeks. Strain out the herbs after this time and bottle the resulting tonic. Take 1 tsp (5 ml) once or twice a day as a recuperative tonic when recovering from illness.

# Valerian
## *Valeriana officinalis*

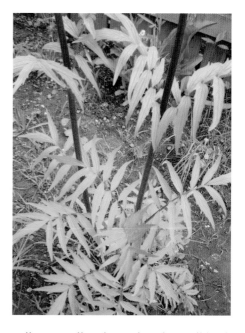

*Also known as:* setwell, amantilla, phew, phu plant, all heal, heliotrope, bouncing bees, pretty betsy, herb of witches, graveyard dust, vandal root, bloody butcher

**Family** Caprifoliaceae.

**Habitat and description** Fantastically statuesque and fragrant, valerian is a fairly common medicinal herb-garden plant, but I have also found it growing wild by rivers and streams, as it does seem to like having its feet wet – in a drought, valerian is often the plant that will wilt first. It has thrived pretty much wherever I have planted it, and self-seeds readily. The plant begins as tender leaves with indented veins – often with a reddish-purple tone – arranged in pairs down a stalk, with a single leaf at the very tip. These leaves turn green as they mature, creating a basal rosette and cluster of leaves in April.

In late May and June, the plant produces incredibly scented flowers that are white and pink, in umbels held well above the basal rosette of leaves – flowers that bees adore, as do the ants often found clambering around the tops of the plants. The root, which can be dug up in autumn and early spring, is thread-like and a real nuisance to clean, but once it is cleaned, it is strong-smelling with that distinctive valerian scent. Cats love the smell of it, so be warned – if you have cats and have some valerian in your home for processing, expect to be very popular, as it has a similar effect on them to catnip!

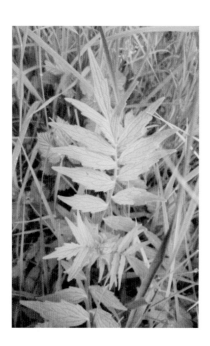

**Where to find it**    Britain, Europe and most temperate regions, including North America.

**Parts used**    Roots.

**When to gather**    Late autumn, winter and early spring.

**Medicines to make**    Aromatic waters, syrups, tinctures, elixirs and teas.

**Constituents**    Iridoid alkaloids known as valpotriates, which are sedative; flavonoids, tannins and essential oils (which your cats will love if they get a whiff of it); sesquiterpenes; gum; resin; sterols.

**Planetary influence**    Mercury.

**Associated deities and heroes**    I suspect trickster Gods, plus those associated with sleep.

**Festival**    Midsummer.

**Constitution**    Hot and dry.

**Actions and indications**    Valerian is a sedative and anxiolytic, making it a useful herb to help relieve stress and anxiety, as well as headaches associated with stress where muscle tension is causing or worsening the problem. Linked issues include nervous stomach ache, palpitations and stomach cramp, all of which valerian can also help with. The root has been used to relieve insomnia and encourage restful sleep, a use of valerian that you'll find pops up a lot in over-the-counter medications. Valerian can also be used to relieve depression that follows excessive anxiety, neuralgia and panic. If you get on well with the herb, it may be a handy thing to include in a panic-attack mix, but make sure you have tried it in drop doses first before you add it to a blend.

As an antispasmodic, it can be used to relieve rheumatic pain, as well as any kind of spasmodic, twisting pain such as intestinal cramp and spasm, colic and wind, as well as period pain and spasms in the bladder and uterus.

Valerian also has some links to the heart and can be used to relieve stress-induced high blood pressure and to slow and strengthen the heart.

One issue with valerian that is important to mention is that in some people it can have a negative reaction, causing mania rather than the relief of anxiety and insomnia. This has happened a few times to my friends and acquaintances, and while some sources suggest that this is due to a release of nervous tension, I have found that it is likely to happen to those who run hot – so if you are prone to a temper and a hot face, have a fast metabolism and a red tongue, and feel the heat easily, you may want to be rather careful if you want to use this herb. Try tiny doses first and work up to larger ones if you need them.

**Folklore**    Valerian has a long history of use, dating from Hippocrates in the fourth century CE. The Anglo-Saxons used it both as a vegetable and as a medicine, and in the Middle Ages it was used as a perfume and a spice – which is interesting, given that most people consider the smell unpleasant (hence the name phu plant!)

It has often been used in the past as a love charm, in potions and spells. The powdered root is known as "graveyard dust" in Voodoo charms, and a related species has been found in Native American warriors' medicine bags, as they used it to heal cuts and wounds.

Cats and rats love the smell of it (I have known of bags of tea shredded by clients' pet cats because the tea had valerian in it!). According to some versions of the Pied Piper story, the Piper himself carried valerian, and the herb is what drew the rats and cats out of Hamelin, not just his pipe music.

**Dose**    2 tsp (10 ml) a day. Go for a cottage tincture for the dosage – a basic tincture of the root steeped in brandy and then strained. If you are buying-in a tincture, 1:3 40% would work fine.

**Contraindications**    I tend to suggest using this with extreme caution in anyone who runs hot, as I have noticed that the tendency to have a bad reaction to valerian seems to be linked with heat excesses. Try a tiny dose to start off with – a dab on the end of the finger should be enough. Monitor how you feel after an hour or two, just to make sure you don't have the negative reaction that sometimes occurs. Extended use of valerian can cause somnolence during the day – not ideal if you have to drive. Using this herb for periods of longer than three months can cause addiction – this is a herb for short-term use only.

# Valerian recipes

## Warming stomach elixir

**Ingredients**
- » 1 tbsp of finely chopped valerian roots
- » 2 tbsp of agrimony leaves
- » 2 tbsp of finely chopped herb bennet roots
- » brandy
- » maple syrup or honey

**Instructions**    As with many elixirs, finely chop the ingredients and pile them into a jar, then pour over enough brandy to just cover the herbs, adding enough honey or syrup to sweeten the mix a little. Let it infuse for a fortnight, then strain out the herbs and bottle the elixir, labelling it for storage. This elixir can help to remedy a sluggish, impaired digestive system that is prone to nausea, wind and bloating after meals and produces too much phlegm. Take 1 tsp (5 ml) twice a day for a fortnight.

## *Sleep elixir*

**Ingredients**
- » 1 tbsp of chopped valerian roots
- » 1 loose handful of mullein flowers
- » 1 tbsp of wood betony leaves
- » 1 handful of chamomile flowers
- » 2 tbsp of chopped lemon balm leaves
- » brandy or vodka
- » honey

**Instructions**    Make sure all the ingredients are thoroughly chopped, and pile them into a clean jar. Pour over enough alcohol to cover the plant matter, and add a spoonful of honey, then let it infuse for a fortnight, shaking it up every other day. Strain out the herbs after this time and bottle the elixir. Take 1 tsp (5 ml) in the evening an hour before bed, to wind down. You can also take ½ tsp (2.5 ml) to calm mid-afternoon stress, but use this cautiously if it makes you sleepy.

# Willow
## *Salix alba*

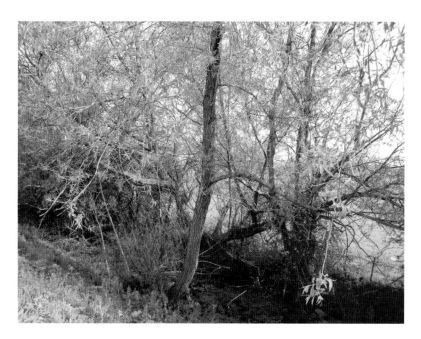

*Also known as:*  osier, pussy willow, saille, salicin willow, saugh tree, tree of enchantment, white willow, withe, withy, witches aspirin, tree of witcheries, sally, welig (Anglo-Saxon, meaning supple)

**Family**  Salicaceae.

**Habitat and description**  The willow tree grows up to heights of 24 m (80 ft) and much prefers to grow near water, although willows can be found growing in less waterlogged soil – I have often seen them growing near natural dew ponds, and also in gardens. Willow is regularly pollarded, as the young branches are used for many different purposes, including basket-making. The bark of the mature tree is gnarled and thick, with deep grooves running vertically down the trunk, and the tree often tends to fork at the base into two heavy trunks. The younger branches have brilliant yellow-green bark with small nodules, and on closer inspection the bark has extremely fine silver lines running vertically down it, possibly the precursor of the fissures found on the adult tree.

Willow leaves are lanceolate, finely serrated at the edges, with fine veins running throughout the leaf, and look very beautiful in the wind. The colour of each leaf is green on top with a silver-coloured underside, turning to yellow gold in the autumn. The tree flowers in May, producing male and female catkins on separate trees. Willow is very easily rooted from the green twigs and is often used to create green sculptures in the garden, as well as living willow arches and fences.

**Where to find it**   Native to Europe and parts of Asia and Africa. Can be found in many temperate regions of the world.

**Parts used**   Bark, leaves.

**When to gather**   Year round for the bark – I recommend mostly taking twigs rather than damaging the main trunk; leaves in late spring.

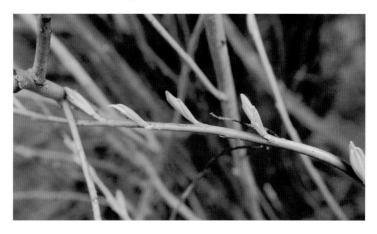

**Medicines to make**   Willow bark tincture, elixir, infused oil and balm; plaisters; washes and baths; decoctions and teas.

**Constituents**   Willow is known for its salicylic acid content, as one of the precursors of modern aspirin. It contains the phenolic glycosides salicin, picein and triandrin, with esters of salicylic acid and salicyl alcohol, acetylated salicin, salicortin and salireposide, as well as tannins, catechin, p-coumaric acid and flavonoids.

**Planetary influence**   The Moon. The tree is essentially feminine in nature, and is ruled by water.

**Associated deities and heroes**   Moon Goddesses in general, the Triple Goddess, most of the witch Goddesses including Hecate and Ceridwen, as well as Persephone, Artemis, Ceres, Brighid and Circe.

**Festival**   Beltane, Samhain.

**Constitution**   Cool and dry.

**Actions and indications**   Culpeper used the plant to stop bleeding from wounds and injuries, as well as to stop any other blood loss, including nose and mouth bleeding and spitting of blood. In his herbal, he also mentioned that it can be used as an anaphrodisiac, although he may have been referring to black willow (*Salix nigra*), as there seems to be some confusion over which variety of willow has this property. Culpeper also used it as a diuretic and the sap to treat eye problems.

Traditionally, willow bark has a long history of use for the treatment of coughs, colds and influenza, as it acts as a febrifuge when drunk hot as well as relieving the discomfort associated with the common cold or flu. A decoction of the bark or a tea of the leaves has also long been used to relieve pain and headaches, and a tea of the leaves can ease colicky type pain in adults.

Willow can also be used to ease a variety of disorders affecting the stomach and digestive system. As it is gently bitter, it can be used as a mild tonic to encourage a better appetite and better liver function, and also to relieve diarrhoea when this is caused by heat and over-relaxed, boggy tissues. Drunk as a tea or decoction, it can ease indigestion and reduce stomach acid; it reduces infection, heat and inflammation, so is potentially a useful ally in relieving food poisoning.

As an extension of its painkilling abilities, it can also be used topically and internally to relieve musculoskeletal complaints such as rheumatism and arthritis, plus inflamed tissues, gout, lumbago, sciatica and neuralgia, acting as both a painkiller and an anti-inflammatory. Use it as a tincture or decoction internally for these properties, or make a strong decoction and add it to the bath water. An infused balm of willow bark may also be a handy addition to the medicine cupboard.

Externally, its astringent properties make it useful in the treatment of ulcers and leucorrhoea, and it has also been used as a scalp tonic to encourage hair growth. A strong tea made with the leaves can be used as a rinse for dandruff. A hot bath made from the bark can be used to treat aches, pains and fevers. Topically, it can be used as a balm to ease sore muscles, aches and pains, and also as a wound healer for cuts, grazes, ulcers and eczema.

**Folklore**    As with most native British trees, there is a wide body of folklore surrounding the willow. It has long had a reputation as a tree of dreams and enchantments, as the name "tree of witcheries" shows. Several of the more famous witches of legend, such as Circe, lived in groves of willow trees. Persephone's grove of willow trees gave the gift of eloquence to Orpheus when he touched the trees growing there – the tree has long had an association with the bardic arts as a result.

Following the tree's long link with witchcraft, the binding on a witch's traditional besom is made from willow withies, in homage to Hecate, the renowned Witch Goddess of legend.

Many of the Sun Gods of myth and legend are associated with the willow and the Moon Goddess – for example, the willow tree that grew outside the cave where Zeus was born, or the willow frame of the coracle the Celtic Sun God Belinos was lifted from as a child. Burial mounds near water are often lined with willow trees, possibly due to the link with Underworld deities. Bearing in mind willow's long link with water and water's long link with the Underworld and the Tree of Life, it comes as no great surprise that the tree is often considered a sacred link between life and death.

An old Celtic tradition of tying cloths and ribbons to willow trees growing near wells and sacred fountains continues to this day.

It is thought that the origin of the saying "knock on wood" derived from the practice of knocking on the willow tree in passing for good fortune. Circe's willow tree grove was part of her sacred cemetery, where male corpses were wrapped in uncured ox skins and left in the tops of willow trees, where the elements might reclaim them. Persephone's grove grew in the far west of Tartarus, another name for the Underworld, further demonstrating the great ties between the willow tree and the Underworld. The Celtic bards and poets thought that "willow tree inspiration" was often preferable to wine or trance in encouraging poetry and eloquence. The bards would sit under the willow trees and listen to the sound of the wind in the tree branches and leaves, and this would encourage the birth of poetry.

**Dose**  5 ml of a tincture or 1 tsp of the bark decocted in a cup of hot water and drunk up to three times a day.

**Contraindications**  Overdosing can cause internal bleeding and excitability. Use willow with caution during pregnancy as well as in cases of gout – salicylic acid can often make gout worse due to increasing the amount of uric acid in the blood.

# Willow recipes

## Willow leaf hair rinse for dandruff

**Ingredients**
- » 1 pint, loosely packed, of willow leaves
- » 570 ml (20 fl oz) of water
- » essential oil, such as lavender or peppermint (optional)

**Instructions**    This is very simple to make. Just roughly chop or shred the leaves and pop them into a saucepan with the water, then bring to a gentle simmer. Simmer for a few minutes, and let it cool with the leaves still in, then strain out the leaves. You can add a couple of drops of essential oil if you want to – lavender or peppermint work really well. Pour into a bottle and use as a rinse after washing your hair.

## Willow cider vinegar hair rinse

**Ingredients**
- » 1 pint, loosely packed, of willow leaves
- » 570 ml (20 fl oz) of cider vinegar, with the mother still in
- » flower water: orange flower, rose, frankincense, or chamomile works well
- » essential oils – peppermint and lavender

**Instructions**    Finely chop the leaves and pack them into a Kilner jar, then pour over plenty of cider vinegar. Let it steep for at least a week, then strain out the herbs and add an equal proportion of flower water to the vinegar. Mix in the essential oils – 10 drops of each per 500 ml (17½ fl oz) of liquid is a good place to start. I tend not to put loads of essential oils into anything that might go near the eyes, so start low and work up from there. Shake the mixture well and use it as a rinse after you wash your hair – make sure it is well massaged into the scalp. Rinse with plenty of warm water. This can improve the condition of the hair and the overall health of the scalp, and may help if the simpler infusion of leaves is not sufficient to deal with scalp issues.

## Willow bark decoction

**Ingredients**
- » 1 tbsp of chopped willow bark
- » 300 ml (10 fl oz) of water

**Instructions**   Make sure the bark is chopped as finely as you can – using bark from fresh twigs is a good idea, as this is much easier to prepare (as described in the Introduction). Put the bark and water into a saucepan, cover with a lid, and put it on a low heat, allowing it to simmer. A simple decoction for lowering fevers probably only needs around half an hour. Strain out the bark and sip the simple decoction in half-mug doses up to three times a day, drunk as hot as you can bear, in order to lower a fever, ease a cold or the flu, or relieve a headache. For a long decoction, which has a much longer shelf life, let it simmer for up to four hours, topping it up with more water as needed. The long decoction is used in much the same way as the short decoction but, as it is stronger, only take doses of 1 tbsp (15 ml) up to four times a day.

## Willow leaf or bark tincture

**Ingredients**
- » 1 pint of leaves or fresh bark
- » 1 bottle of vodka or brandy
- » honey, if you want to make an elixir

**Instructions**   If you are using leaves, finely chop them and pack them into a Kilner jar, pouring over the alcohol and adding the honey if you want to use it. Put the lid on and let it sit for at least a fortnight, shaking regularly. This being willow, you might consider making it on the full moon and leaving it until the following full moon.

If you are using bark, chop it as much as you can and pack it into a Kilner jar, then repeat the same process as with the leaves. Bark can be more of a nuisance to work with – if it is really tough, consider boiling up a slow decoction and preserving that with the alcohol. Once filtered, take 1 tsp (5 ml) of the leaf or bark tincture three times a day.

## Willow bark-and-leaf infused oil

**Ingredients**

- » roughly chopped fresh willow bark and leaves (if using them)
- » organic oil: rapeseed, sunflower, sweet almond or olive all work well

**Instructions**    You can use leaves or bark or a combination of both for this recipe, depending on what you have to hand. Chop or shred the leaves and/or bark as much as you can and pile them into a double boiler with the oil, bringing the water in the lower pan to a simmer. Let it simmer for at least an hour. Strain and repeat the process with fresh plant matter, to make a stronger oil. If you are using bark as well as leaves, it will need to steep for longer to pull the medicinal properties out of the tougher bark surface. You could infuse the bark first, possibly in a slow cooker with the oil, then strain out the spent bark and compost it, and repeat the process using chopped leaves. Once you are happy with your infused oil, pour the whole lot through a piece of kitchen towel into a bowl or jug and let it sit for a while to allow any water to sink to the bottom. If you are making the balm in the following recipe, measure out 100 ml (3½ fl oz) of the oil and reserve – bottle the rest and label it with the date, English and Latin names and its uses. The oil can be used as a bath oil or as a muscle rub or massage oil; it can also be made into a balm or ointment.

## Willow bark-and-leaf infused balm

### Ingredients
» 100 ml (3½ fl oz) of willow bark-and-leaf infused oil (previous recipe)
» 10 g of beeswax
» 20 drops of essential oil of your choice, such as frankincense, peppermint, rosemary or lavender

**Instructions**   Pour the willow bark-and-leaf infused oil into the top of the double boiler (making sure any remaining bits of leaf and bark from the infusing process have been filtered out), and add the beeswax. Bring to a gentle simmer and stir occasionally until the beeswax has melted, then stir in the essential oils and pour the balm into jars. Once slightly cooled, lid the jars to stop the essential oils from evaporating. Use this balm for sore joints, aches and pains. You can add 40 drops of lavender essential oil to the final recipe and rub the mixture onto the back of the neck and the temples, to ease headaches.

You can also pour this balm onto a clean tea towel and bandage it onto sore joints to relieve the pain of sports injuries, rheumatism and arthritis.

# Wood sage
## *Teucrium scorodonia*

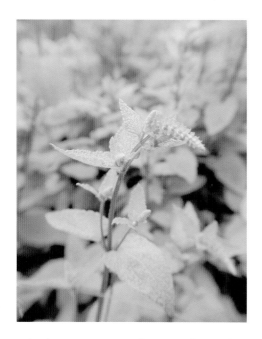

*Also known as:*   wood germander, garlic sage

**Family**   Lamiaceae.

**Habitat and description**   A fairly typical member of the mint family, wood sage forms clumps of growth in shady areas, though it will also happily grow in full sun. It seems to prefer well-drained soil – I have found it growing wild on chalk cliffs overhanging the sea, as well as in woodlands, meadows and other areas, including my herb garden, which ranges from full sun to full shade. The plant itself isn't tremendously tall, only reaching a height of around 65 cm (25 in.) at full growth, and it features rounded, roughly triangular leaves in opposite pairs up a square stem. The flowers in summer are pale green and quite small – beautiful when observed closely but easily overlooked. They are, however, much beloved by bees and insects, and lead to pale-brown seed heads filled with seeds that self sow readily. The leaves of the plant are aromatic when crushed, with a fragrance that is reminiscent of sage, thyme and marjoram – all members of the same plant family.

**Where to find it**    Native to Western Europe including the UK, but has since naturalised to other parts of the world including North America and New Zealand.

**Parts used**    Aerial parts.

**When to gather**    Late summer and autumn.

**Medicines to make**    Infused oils, salves and ointments, teas, decoctions, elixirs and tinctures, skin washes.

**Constituents**    Tannins and essential oils, diterpenes, iridoids and flavonoids; pyrrolizidine alkaloids.

**Planetary influence**    Venus.

**Associated deities and heroes**    None known at present.

**Festival**    None known at present.

**Constitution**    Cold and dry.

**Actions and indications**    Wood sage is no longer widely used in herbal medicine, as the presence of liver-toxic pyrrolizidine alkaloids has been detected. As with many herbs, this does make the plant a little more tricky to use, but bear in mind that not all herbs are tonics, and such is certainly the case with this plant. Wood sage is for short-term use only, for specific health complaints, and I advise avoiding it totally if you have any history of liver issues – better safe than sorry, after all. That having been said, the plant has a range of useful properties, including being stimulant and antiseptic, anticatarrhal and anti-inflammatory, making it very useful for treating chest infections, bronchitis, and colds in general, especially where a large amount of phlegm and pulmonary inflammation is present. It will help the body to sweat out a fever when drunk as a hot tea, as well as helping the body to excrete excess amounts of phlegm and mucus.

The herb is also a bitter digestive tonic, providing carminative properties for those with poor digestion and appetite, where food intake results in wind, griping and bloating. It has some nervine actions, particularly where the nerves are strung taut due to overwork and exhaustion – again, for short-term use only. Consider using it for a week, then trading it for two weeks with a less potentially troublesome herb for the digestion, such as agrimony, fennel or sweet cicely.

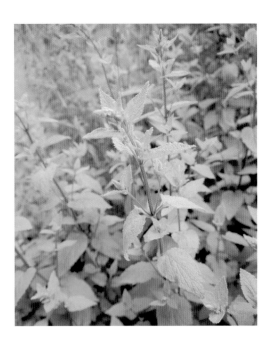

Topically, the herb really comes into its own, making an excellent spray for cuts and grazes, wounds that refuse to heal or are seeping pus, as well as for sores and ulcers. Combine it with yarrow for this purpose, or just use it on its own, either as an alcohol-based infusion or as a water-infused skin wash.

**Folklore**　　Wood sage is used instead of hops as a beer flavouring in some parts of the world, though it imparts a different colour to the finished brew. It apparently makes beer clear faster than hops do.

**Dose**　　This varies considerably, but up to 10 ml a day of the tincture works well (but see Contraindications).

**Contraindications**　　Wood sage contains pyrrolizidine alkaloids, which are toxic to the liver in large quantities. Use it internally with caution, by only taking small doses for no more than two weeks at a time. Avoid it totally if you have any liver issues.

# Wood sage recipes

## Wood sage and yarrow wound spray

**Ingredients**
- » 1 large handful of wood sage
- » 1 large handful of yarrow flowering tops
- » vodka

**Instructions**　　Finely chop the herbs and pile them into a Kilner jar, then pour over enough vodka to cover the herbs, with an extra couple of centimetres on top. Put the lid on and shake it up every other day, leaving the whole lot to infuse for at least a fortnight, then strain the herbs through a coffee filter paper before bottling it into a spray bottle. This can be sprayed onto cuts, wounds, suppurating ulcers and any other open cut, graze or wound, to kill any bacteria and encourage healing.

## Wood sage, thyme and lemon tea

**Ingredients**
- » 1 tsp of chopped fresh wood sage and thyme leaves
- » ½ lemon, sliced
- » hot water
- » honey, sugar or maple syrup (if preferred)

**Instructions**    Pile the wood sage, thyme and lemon into a large mug, teapot or cafetiere and pour over one mug of hot water, just off the boil. Cover the cup and let it steep for 5 minutes, then strain out the herbs, add honey, sugar or maple syrup to taste, and drink hot. This will encourage the body to get rid of excess pulmonary phlegm, as well as easing chest infections and bronchitis. Drink one cup twice a day. If you're running a fever as well as having a chest infection, add in some elderflower, or replace the thyme with elderflower.

# Wormwood
## *Artemisia absinthium*

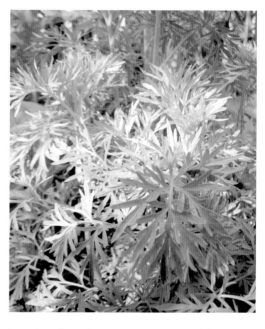

*Also known as:* absinthe, absinthium, green ginger, old woman, crown for a king, madderwort, wormot

**Family**  Asteraceae.

**Habitat and description**  Wormwood is a perennial; it reaches heights of around 1 m (3 ft), growing quite happily in tubs or in the herb garden. It has deeply lobed leaves that are a silvery green in colour, slightly more silver than green on the undersides, with tiny silvery-yellow flowers. The leaves are covered with very fine, silky hairs, and the whole plant has a familiar aromatic fragrance that is very deceptive – it smells as if it should taste quite good, but the whole plant is unpleasantly bitter.

It can be grown from seed, though it is also possible to take stem cuttings during the summer. Prune plants in the late autumn – they tend to die back around about then anyway, so that usually reminds me to do the job. Wormwood is not a good neighbour to sage, fennel, anise or caraway – don't plant it next to these four plants, as it will inhibit their growth. I find wormwood is quite a bully and will crowd out lower-growing plants, so best to grow it at the back of the border and give it plenty of space to stretch out, or risk losing some of the denizens of your herb garden. It will self-seed quite readily, given half a chance.

**Where to find it**   Wormwood is native to Europe; it will grow quite happily in the UK, as long as it has plenty of sunlight and reasonably dry, well-drained soil. It can be found in most temperate zones of the world, as well as in

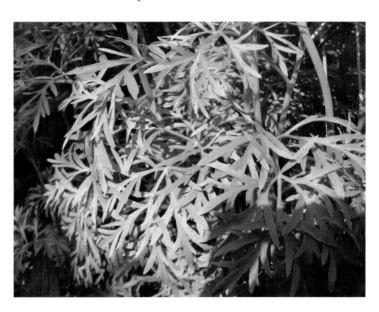

Northern Africa, and it has naturalised in parts of North America and India.

**Parts used**   Aerial parts, roots.

**When to gather**   Summer through autumn.

**Medicines to make**   Digestive bitters; tinctures; infused oils (for topical use only); smudge sticks; aromatic waters; root tincture.

**Constituents**   Volatile oils consisting of alpha and beta thujone; azulenes such as chamazulene; sesquiterpene lactones, including absinthin, artemetin and isoabsinthin; acetylines in the root; flavonoids such as quercetin-3-glucosides; phenolic acids such as vanillic and syringic acids; and, lastly, lignans.

**Planetary influence**   Mars.

**Associated deities and heroes**   Diana, Artemis, Aesculapius, Horus, Isis.

**Festival**   I suspect probably Samhain, because of its association with scrying and divination. It is also associated with Imbolc.

**Constitution**   Hot and dry.

**Actions and indications**   Due to its intensely bitter taste, wormwood is often used as a digestive bitter and as a stomachic and choleretic. It has some anti-inflammatory properties due to the presence of chamazulenes and so can be used for inflammatory digestive disorders. It is used to treat liver and gall bladder congestion where this has led to jaundice, as well as liver-related depression, lack of appetite, nausea and vomiting. As it is warming, it is particularly good for those who suffer from a depressed autonomic nervous system, leading to impaired digestive function. Additionally, it can be used to treat diarrhoea and intestinal parasites.

Wormwood can be used in cases of nervous exhaustion and other nerve issues, such as neuralgia and depression. It can apparently be used to ease alcohol-induced hangovers – though a better bet, in my opinion, would be to dose up on milk thistle before starting to drink or simply not drink as much. (I know, boring solution, but eminently practical!) This is another of those odd herbs with a dual nature, like Valerian mentioned earlier, which can sometimes cause the very symptoms it is supposed to treat. Wormwood can be used to ameliorate the effects of epilepsy, but it will also cause seizures if you use it in large enough doses – making me wonder whether this plant has some ties with Mercury, as this dual nature often occurs in plants linked with this tricky planet.

Wormwood has a strong antibacterial property – the root, though not often used in medicine, is extremely powerful and useful in easing infections of the throat and lungs. It helps to relieve pain and is very cooling and soothing – unusual, given that the rest of the plant is considered to be heating. It can be used topically as an antiseptic.

As an emmenagogue, it can be used to stimulate absent menses where this is due to uterine stagnation, which causes delayed menstruation. It can also be used to ease painful periods. It is used as a pain reliever during labour and can be taken as a weak tea or applied as a rub to stimulate sluggish labour, when contractions are too weak.

A rub made with the essential oil can be used to relieve the pain of arthritis and related joint complaints, though the oil must NEVER be taken internally.

It can also be used to ease benzodiazepine withdrawal for those who have become addicted to it. The leaf can be used as an infusion against malaria, as it inhibits the disease. It is extremely useful in the treatment of antibiotic-resistant disease and deserves a much better reputation than it already has. However, this herb must be used cautiously by the layperson, as the thujone content is poisonous and can be damaging in large doses.

**Folklore**    Most people with an interest in herbs will be well aware that wormwood is the main ingredient of the infamous drink known as absinthe, *la fée vert* or the green fairy, so beloved of artists, muses and general alcoholics of the Victorian era, especially in France. Absinthe is highly addictive and can cause insanity in large enough doses – Van Gogh cut off his own ear under the influence of absinthe. This rather puts me in mind of the old legend concerning spending the night on certain mountains, whereby the pilgrim would return either mad or a poet – I rather suspect absinthe draws certain parallels with the mountain. If taken by someone with a certain amount of mental fragility, it will crack the mind wide open and can induce cracks in the mind of even the strongest person if taken in large enough or frequent enough doses. In small doses, however, it is reputed to free poetry from the mind – rather a risky undertaking, if you ask me, especially considering that these days absinthe is illegal in most parts of the world. Much better to use a drop dose of the weak wormwood tincture instead.

Wormwood's Latin name of *Artemisia* is, quite obviously, named for Artemis, Goddess of the Moon and the Hunt – appropriate enough, given some of our words for madness, such as lunacy, moon mad or moon struck; a fitting name for a plant that can be used to induce madness.

Apparently wormwood marked the path the serpent took when it was kicked out of Eden. Another legend tells that wormwood was given by Diana to the centaur Chiron, the famous healer of myth. Later folklore links the plant with the Mexican salt Goddess: women wore garlands of the herb on their heads during the ceremonial dance to celebrate the Goddess.

**Dose**    No more than 4 ml three times per day, or 1 tsp of the dried herb in a cup of hot water drunk three times a day. The remedy is so bitter that you probably won't want to drink a tea of it, however.

**Contraindications**    Not safe during pregnancy or while breast-feeding. The thujone content is poisonous in large doses, so if you are going to use this herb, use it with extreme caution and respect and exclusively in drop doses.

# Wormwood recipes

## Wormwood bitters

**Ingredients**
- » 1 large bunch of fresh wormwood leaves
- » 1 orange
- » 1 tsp of fennel seeds
- » 1 piece of sweet cicely root (optional)
- » vodka

**Instructions**    Finely chop the leaves and pile them into a jar, and add the zest of the orange, also finely chopped, as this has its own properties that ease griping and stomach cramps. Bash up the fennel seeds using a mortar and pestle and add them to the jar, and finely chop and add the sweet cicely, if you are using it, then pour over enough vodka to cover the herbs. Put the lid on and shake it up every other day, leaving it to steep for a month; then strain out the herbs and put some of the resulting bitters into a dropper bottle. Take 1–3 drops half an hour before a meal to stimulate the appetite and act as a tonic for the digestion. Do not sweeten this recipe – bitters need to act on the vagus nerve in order to stimulate the proper flow of digestive enzymes.

## Wormwood smudge sticks

**Ingredients / equipment**
- » plenty of fresh wormwood leaves
- » cotton yarn

**Instructions**   Make sure the leaves are clean and dry to the touch, then cut the stems into 20-cm (8-in.) lengths and pile them up in groups of up to ten stems, turning each stem added to face the opposite direction to the one before it. Once you have a bundle that is a good 2.5 cm (1 in.) thick, cut a long piece of yarn – at least a metre (3¼ ft). Wrap one end of it four or five times around one end of the bundle, pulling it tight, then tie it off, leaving one long trailing end as well as the remainder of the yarn. Wrap the yarn around and down the bundle, pulling it firmly around the herbs, and repeat the process at the other end, pulling the thread tight as you wrap it several times around the herbs. Wrap the rest of the yarn back up the bundle to the top, and tie it off to the trailing end left earlier. Lay the finished smudge sticks out on a tray to dry slowly. These can be lit and then blown out, and the smoke can be used to smudge persons, items or places. Smudging is the use of smoke to remove negative influences from the air – be they smell, bacteria or viruses, or energy. Smudging is a Native American practice, but I believe the Anglo-Saxons also used a form of it for similar purposes.

## Wormwood-and-rosemary infused oil

**Ingredients**
- » plenty of fresh wormwood leaves
- » several sprigs of fresh rosemary
- » organic seed oil
- » warming essential oils, such as ginger, black pepper, ravensara etc.

**Instructions**    Finely chop the clean, surface-dry leaves and pile them into a slow cooker if you have one, or into a double boiler if not. Pour over enough organic seed oil to cover the leaves, then put the slow cooker on the low setting and leave it for several hours, or overnight if possible. This long, slow infusion will encourage the more resiny rosemary to begin to extract into the oil. You can repeat the process with fresh herbs the following day. Once you are happy with the strength of the oil, strain out the herbs and add 5 drops of your chosen essential oils per 100 ml (3½ fl oz) of oil. Shake it up vigorously. This can be massaged thoroughly into sore muscles and arthritic joints, to warm them and relieve inflammation.

# Yarrow
## *Achillea millefolium*

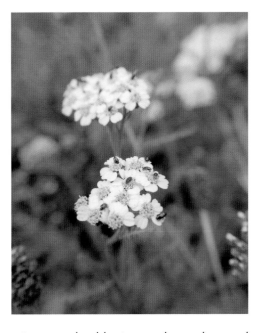

*Also known as:* old man's mustard, soldier's woundwort, thousand seal, milfoil, arrow root, wound wort, devil's bit, snake grass, death flower, seven year's love, military herb, knight's milfoil, field hops, devil's plaything, ladies' mantle, nosebleed, knyghten, eerie, devil's nettle, staunch, stench grass, gris, yarroway, old man's pepper, sanguinary, sneezewort, bloodwort, thousand leaf

**Family**   Asteraceae.

**Habitat and description**   Yarrow grows on wasteland and in hedges, gardens, fields, meadows and woodland – in short, most places where plants can grow. It likes sun but will grow in shade. While it prefers a rich, moist soil, that is not the best ground for growing the most aromatic yarrow – this can be found on scrubby wasteland, where it has had to work somewhat harder for its survival. The plant usually has a basal rosette of feathery, deeply divided leaves from which its Latin name "*millefolium*" derives, out of which rise tall stems of white or sometimes pale-pink flowers, each of which has five small petals. The plant grows up to a height of 90 cm (about 3 feet) and flowers in late summer and early autumn, the preferred time for collecting the plant matter.

**Where to find it**    Yarrow is a familiar sight throughout the UK and Europe and is also found widely in North America and elsewhere.

**Parts used**    The whole plant is used in herbal medicine.

**When to gather**    When the plant is in flower, in August and September.

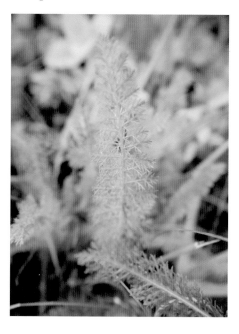

**Medicines to make**   Teas, tinctures, liqueurs and elixirs; infused oils, balms and skin washes.

**Constituents**   Volatile oil, including azulenes such as camazulene; also sesquiterpenes and sesquiterpene lactones, flavonoids, alkaloids and bases, and salicylic acid.

**Planetary influence**   Venus.

**Associated deities and heroes**   Woodland deities – Cernunnos, Herne and Pan.

**Festival**   Lughnasadh / Lammas.

**Constitution**   Temperate and dry.

**Actions and indications**   Yarrow has a wide variety of actions and indications, and while it is best known for its vulnerary action, making it a useful remedy for cuts and wounds, it also has plenty of other uses.

Renowned herbalist Nicholas Culpeper was of the opinion that yarrow is drying and binding, and astringent in nature, used for the "flux", for green wounds, ulcers and fistulas, as well as "staying the shedding of hair, the head being bathed with the decoction of it". He reckoned it was useful for some reproductive disorders, such as leucorrhoea, and for gonorrhoea, and he commented that it makes a useful ointment for wounds.

Generally speaking, these days it is used as a circulatory herb, and is brilliant for toning up the blood vessels. It supports healthy circulation around the body and can be used alongside herbs such as hawthorn to help relieve slightly elevated blood pressure. As a vasotonic alterative, it improves the tone of veins and the peripheral circulation, making it useful for anyone suffering from cold hands and feet, including those with Raynaud's disease. Its use is also beneficial in cases of thrombosis and varicose veins.

Yarrow is anti-inflammatory and diuretic, which makes it very helpful, when combined with herbs such as burdock or cleavers, for assisting the removal of toxins around the joints that can cause worsening of rheumatism.

As a diaphoretic, it makes a superb remedy to relieve influenza and feverish disorders, as it helps the body to break out in a healing sweat and thereby lower its temperature. It is part of the old traditional blend for influenza and related respiratory complaints: two parts each of yarrow and elderflower to one part peppermint.

In addition to the above complaints, it can be used for digestive problems such as dysentery, diarrhoea, IBS and anorexia, and for women's complaints such as amenorrhoea, dysmenorrhoea and menorrhagia. It is particularly useful in the treatment of intermittent fever when taken as a hot infusion, as it stimulates sweating. As a cold infusion, it tones the mucous membranes and stimulates the appetite. Drinking too much yarrow can bring on a bone-deep chill, as it moves the heat outwards – as I discovered while drinking it when on the mend after a bout of food poisoning: I drank a large amount of the warm infusion and spent the next two hours with bone-deep, shaking cold.

Externally, yarrow is superb for cuts and trauma bruises, where it dries up and tones the blood vessels, stops bleeding and disperses blood under the skin. It makes a great balm for martial artists and those who can clearly remember where and how they got that bruise.

**Folklore**   The name "*Achillea*" means "herb of Achilles". The centaur Chiron taught Achilles how to use yarrow to treat his and his soldiers' wounds in battle. The name "*millefolium*" refers to the feathery leaves. Yarrow has many different folk names, most of which refer to its use to treat wounds and stop bleeding. Yarrow has been used by many different civilizations around the world for similar purposes – the healing of wounds, among others, and also to ward off negativity.

During the Middle Ages, it was a herb used by and against witches, as well as to keep evil spirits away from livestock dwellings. The original *I Ching* was composed of yarrow stalks, so it is an excellent divinatory herb.

**Dose**    I recommend using 4 g of the dried herb, 1 tsp (4 ml) of a liquid extract, or 2 tsp (10 ml) of tincture – these are for one-off dosages. A good dosage for infusions is 1 tsp (5 g), heaped, of the dried herb to one cup of boiling water, three times per day for chronic ailments, or every two hours for acute infections. Bear in mind that if you drink it to mop up after food poisoning and related issues, too much of it will make you cold to the very bone!

**Contraindications**    This herb should be avoided during pregnancy, due to the presence of thujone. Large doses can cause headaches.

# Yarrow recipes

## Hawthorn and yarrow tonic

**Ingredients**
- » 500 g (1 lb 1½ oz) of fresh hawthorn berries, or 300 g (10½ oz) of dried berries
- » 1 lemon
- » 5 cm (2 in.) piece of fresh root ginger
- » 4 tbsp, heaped, of dried yarrow flowering tops and leaves
- » brandy or vodka
- » local honey

**Instructions**    Put the hawthorn berries into a Kilner jar – do not crush them first! If you crush them, the high pectin content in the berries usually means that your elixir will set solid and be more of an alcoholic jelly than a liquid; this is definitely a problem if, like me, you originally made this recipe in a fairly narrow-necked jar, as it was impossible to get it out of the pot again! Zest the lemon and chop it finely, then juice it and add the juice and zest to the jar. I also like to add a piece of fresh root ginger to this recipe – chop it finely (into 2 mm-square pieces works well).

Lastly, thoroughly shred the dried yarrow, add it to the jar, and use a long spoon to stir it all up. This recipe could also be made using fresh yarrow instead of dried: if you want to do this, use double the quantity of yarrow stated and chop it as finely as you can. Now pour over plenty of alcohol – you want enough to allow an extra 5 cm (2 in.) on top of the ingredients. Add 2 large tablespoons of local honey, put the lid on, and shake it up thoroughly, then store it in a cool, dark place. Shake the mixture every couple of days and let it steep for at least two weeks – I generally like to leave my berry recipes for more like a month. Filter out the ingredients at the end of this time and take 2 tsp (10 ml) once a day as a tonic. It can make a pleasant-tasting evening drink, either neat or with a little added fruit juice.

If you would prefer not to use alcohol, you can make a version of this with unpasteurised, raw apple cider vinegar instead; this recipe uses exactly the same quantities as listed above, but swaps out the alcohol for vinegar. This can be used in similar doses, but it will need to be mixed with a little water first.

## Yarrow and hawthorn syrup

### Ingredients
» 500 g (1 lb 1½ oz) of fresh hawthorn berries, or 300 g (10½ oz) of dried berries

» 4 tbsp heaped, of dried yarrow flowering tops and leaves
» 1 lemon
» 5 cm (2 in.) piece of fresh root ginger
» 1.2 l (40 fl oz) of water
» 1 kg (2 lb 3½ oz) brown sugar

**Instructions**     Zest and juice the lemon and add it to a pan with the chopped ginger, the hawthorn and yarrow, and the water. Bring to a gentle boil, and let it simmer for at least half an hour, mashing occasionally to break the skins of the hawthorn berries. Once the liquid has turned gently pink and reduced down by a quarter, strain out the herbs and put the liquid back into the pan with the sugar. Bring to a gentle simmer, stirring until the sugar has dissolved, then boil for several minutes, stirring regularly. Take it off the heat after this time and pour it into clean bottles, labelling it clearly. You can take this syrup as a daily medicine by the dessertspoonful (10 ml), or pour it over porridge, pancakes, cakes or puddings, or use as a mixer with an infused vodka or alcohol.

## Yarrow, elder and daisy bruise balm

**Ingredients**
» 1 large handful each of yarrow leaves and flowering tops
» 1 large handful of elder leaves
» 2–3 tbsp of daisy flowers
» organic seed oil
» beeswax
» rosemary and peppermint essential oils

**Instructions**     Thoroughly chop the herbs and infuse them in the seed oil in a double boiler, making sure the oil covers the herbs – allow an extra centimetre of oil on top of the herbs. Let the whole lot steep for at least an hour, then strain out the herbs. Add 12 g of beeswax per 100 ml (3½ fl oz) of infused oil, and return both to the double boiler, warming the mixture through and stirring until the wax has melted. Add 10 drops each of the two essential oils, stir briefly and pour the resulting salve into jars. Put the lid on and let it cool, then label it carefully. This balm is superb for bruises and bumps.

# Additional winter recipes

Due to the rather arbitrary designation of herbs into seasons, some herbs might be classified as summer herbs even though parts of them are better suited to autumn and winter. Below are some extra recipes using herbs that are not covered in this book in detail but that are, nevertheless, eminently worth gathering in autumn and winter for use.

## Nettle golden milk

**Ingredients**
- » plenty of freshly dug nettle roots – around 1 tbsp per person, if possible
- » milk or milk alternative
- » honey or maple syrup
- » cinnamon

**Instructions**    Finely chop the freshly dug and scrubbed nettle root, which should be a golden yellow colour. Pile it into a saucepan and add one mug of milk or milk substitute per person, plus a good pinch of cinnamon per cup, then bring to a gentle simmer and let it steep for 5 minutes before taking it off the heat. Sweeten to taste – I find 1 tsp (5 ml) of honey per cup is usually a pleasant amount, but you can add more if you prefer. Stir, cool slightly, and drink as hot as you can. This is a wonderful tonic for the winter and a perfect remedy for digging the vegetable or herb beds, as you can use some of the nettle root unearthed while stopping the plant's incorrigible push towards world domination!

## Elder and blackberry honey

**Ingredients**
- » ½ pint of fresh elderberries
- » ½ pint of fresh blackberries
- » 330 g jar of local runny honey

**Instructions**   Check over the berries for bird poop or small passengers, and pile the blackberries into a saucepan, adding the elderberries once they have been stripped from their stems. Add 1 tbsp (15 ml) of water and put the pan on a low heat to get the berries to burst and the juices to flow, then cook gently until the berries are thoroughly mashed down. Leave the fruit pulp to cool, then pile it into a sieve and push it through, leaving the seeds behind, before putting the whole lot back into the cleaned pan. Simmer gently until the concoction has reduced by about half. The idea here is to begin working towards creating a rob, but to stop before it thickens too much. The ideal consistency is to get it to the point where you can stir it, scraping the spoon against the bottom of the pan, and the pulp does not rush to refill the line left by the spoon. Once you are happy with the thickness of the concoction, pour in the entire jar of runny honey and stir it in well, then decant the dark mixture back into clean jars, put the lid on and label it. I have found this mixture lasts for easily six months or longer and is a delicious alternative to a sugar-laden syrup. Take 1 tsp (5 ml) twice a day as a prophylactic to ward off the common cold or flu, or use it to spoon over pancakes, stir into teas and infusions, or add to porridge or overnight oats.

## Elderberry and star anise syrup

### Ingredients
- » 20 heads of elderberries or more
- » 2 whole star anise, crushed
- » 1 organic lemon
- » 1 l water
- » 1 kg (2 lb 3½ oz) of brown sugar – preferably organic or Fairtrade

**Instructions**    Strip the berries off the stems and pile them into a saucepan with the water, along with the juice and zest of the lemon and the crushed star anise. You can also add other spices if you want, but I find that star anise on its own gives the syrup a lovely flavour and makes it less dense than the traditional recipe, which usually contains cloves. Bring the pan of water and ingredients to a gentle simmer and cook for half an hour, mashing occasionally to ensure that all the berries have burst and given up their goodness to the water. Strain the mixture through a jelly bag (used in jam making) or muslin cloth and put it back into the cleaned pan with the sugar, then bring the whole lot to a gentle simmer again, stirring until the sugar has dissolved. Now bring the syrup up to a rolling boil and let it cook for 10 minutes, stirring regularly – watch it carefully at this stage, as syrups have the tendency to boil over. Once the syrup has thickened slightly, pour it into clean bottles while it is still hot, put the tops on immediately, and label them carefully. This can be taken daily as a winter tonic or poured over desserts or breakfasts; it should keep for up to six months in a cool cupboard, though I usually find I have given away half of mine before the first winter cold hits!

# Recommended reading

For those wanting to continue their explorations into the ancient healing arts of herbalism, here is a list of books that I thoroughly recommend as being enlightening, inspiring and entertaining to read. This is really just a very brief list – there are so many excellent books out there that I haven't yet stumbled across that I have no doubt the list could easily be three times as long!

*Alchemical Medicine for the 21ˢᵗ Century – Spagyrics for Detox, Healing and Longevity*
Clare Goodrick-Clarke
ISBN 978–1–59477–913–8
This is a superb, accessible guide to making your own spagyric tinctures, written in language that is comprehensive yet approachable. If you want to have a go at this elaborate and fascinating procedure, this book will give you an excellent jumping-off point.

*A Modern Herbal*
Mrs M. Grieve
ISBN 1–90477–901–8
This is one of the grandmothers of herb books, and is an immense tome. Worth getting for any herbal historian.

*A Woman's Book of Herbs*
Elisabeth Brooke
ISBN 978–1–91159–722–3
Beautifully written and inspiring; particularly well suited to those with a more feminist mindset.

*Complete Earth Medicine Handbook*
Susanne Fischer-Rizzi
ISBN 1–40270–430–5
One of the most beautiful herb books I have ever seen – illustrated with whimsical pencil sketches throughout, and covering some of the more unusual herbs, with some fascinating recipes.

*Hedgerow Medicine*
Julie Bruton Seal and Matthew Seal
ISBN 978–1–87367–499–4
Covering many of our more common hedgerow herbs and illustrated with a plethora of beautiful photographs.

*Herb Craft – A Guide to the Shamanic and Ritual Use of Herbs*
Susan Lavender and Anna Franklin
ISBN 1–89830–757–9
If you are interested in the more magical side of plants, this is the book for you.

*Practical Herbs 1 / Practical Herbs 2*
Henriette Kress
ISBN 978–952–67575–0–6 / 978–952–68025–0–3
Henriette Kress has been an internet staple for many a year now, and was definitely an influence when I was first training. These two books of hers are superb – approachable and full of useful information.

*The Earthwise Herbal – A Complete Guide to Old World Medicinal Plants /*
*The Earthwise Herbal – A Complete Guide to New World Medicinal Plants*
Matthew Wood
ISBN 978–1–55643–692–5 / ISBN 978–1–55643–779–3
Matthew Wood needs no real introduction to any herb lover, and his two books are worthy of a place on any herbalist's shelf. Packed full of information, with more specific indications for each plant.

*Evolutionary Herbalism*
> Sajah Boreham
> ISBN 978–1–62317–313–5
> This wonderful book links together a variety of different methods
> for deciding which herbs to use for which physical types, including
> Ayurvedic principles, planetary and astrological principles, and many
> more. A really superb addition to the herb library, and beautifully
> written as well, this book contains too much information to boil down
> to a simple paragraph.

*The Herbal Medicine Maker's Handbook – A Home Manual*
> James Green
> ISBN 978–0–89594–990–5
> A comprehensive guide to an array of different medicine-making
> skills, and written in a highly engaging fashion.

*The Language of Plants – A Guide to the Doctrine of Signatures*
> Julia Graves
> ISBN 978–1–58420–098–7
> For those wanting to gain a more thorough understanding of the
> Doctrine of Signatures and how to use it as a road map, this is an
> excellent book.

*The Medicinal Flora of Britain and Northwestern Europe*
> Julian Barker
> ISBN 1–87458–163–0
> Featuring almost all the wild flowers growing throughout the UK
> and Europe, this is recommended for anyone wanting to gain
> information on some of the more weird and wonderful of our
> medicinal plants.

*Under the Witching Tree*
> Corinne Boyer
> ISBN 978–1–90960–218–2
> Any books by Corinne Boyer are infinitely worth a read if you are
> fascinated by folklore as well as medicine – she writes beautifully, in a
> lyrical style, while still giving plenty of information.

*Weeds in the Heart*
> Nathanial Hughes and Fiona Owen
> ISBN 978–0–99292–182–8
> This is a veritable spellbook of herbs, full of the most stunning illustrations and beautifully written.

*Witchcraft Medicine – Healing Arts, Shamanic Practices and Forbidden Plants*
> Claudia Muller Ebeling, Christian Ratsch and Wolf-Dieter Storl
> ISBN 978–0–89281–971–3
> This book takes your mind places. If you would like to better understand the place of plants for our ancestors, this is a book you may want to delve into.

# Index